SPORTS 2nd edition
SUPPLEMENTS

SPORTS 2nd edition
SUPPLEMENTS

Which Nutritional Supplements Really Work

ANITA BEAN

B L O O M S B U R Y
LONDON · NEW DELHI · NEW YORK · SYDNEY

Note

While every effort has been made to ensure that the content of this book
is as technically accurate and as sound as possible, neither the author nor
the publishers can accept responsibility for any injury or loss sustained as
a result of the use of this material.

Published by Bloomsbury Publishing Plc
50 Bedford Square
London WC1B 3DP
www.bloomsbury.com

Bloomsbury is a trademark of Bloomsbury Publishing plc

Second edition 2015

First edition published in 2007

ISBN (print): 9781472909664
ISBN (epub): 9781472911452
ISBN (epdf): 9781472911582

Acknowledgements

Cover photographs © Shutterstock

Inside photographs © Shutterstock.com with the exception of the following:
p.10 © Niloo/Shutterstock.com; p.30 © Vsevolod33/Shutterstock.com;
p.33 © Natursports/Shutterstock.com; p.46 © Diego Barbien/Shutterstock.com;
p.68 © muratart/Shutterstock.com; pp.74–5 © Mr Pics/Shutterstock.com;
p.104 © Maxisport/Shutterstock.com; p.113 © PhotoStock10/Shutterstock.com;
p.150 © Marcel Jancovic/Shutterstock.com; pp. 60 and 63 © Getty images

Commissioning Editor: Charlotte Croft

Editor: Sarah Cole

Typeset in URW Grotesk Light by seagulls.net

Printed and bound in China by Toppan Lee Fung Printing

10 9 8 7 6 5 4 3 2 1

CONTENTS

INTRODUCTION

Since the publication of the first edition of *Sports Supplements*, the number of pills, potions and supplements promising performance enhancement has continued to grow unabatedly. And we're spending more on them than ever before. Globally, the market was worth $20.7 billion in 2012 and is forecast to reach $37.7 billion in 2019*. It seems that sports supplements are no longer only the domain of bodybuilders and hard-core athletes; they are now sold in supermarkets and high street shops, as well as gyms, health stores and through the internet. They have become mainstream.

The trouble is, with the multitude of products on the market, separating hype and fact isn't easy. Many supplements are advertised alongside impressive testimonials or celebrity endorsements, which can make the product's claims appear very convincing. Manufacturers often promise dramatic results, pepper their adverts with technical jargon and cite studies cherry-picked to back their claims. All this makes it difficult to know the truth about a product and whether it really works.

What's more, there is no systematic regulation of sports supplements, which means there's no guarantee that a supplement lives up to its claims or doesn't contain banned substances. Most sports organisations, including the International Olympic Committee (IOC), UK Sport, and the US National Collegiate Athletic Association (NCAA) have developed policies on sports supplements and caution athletes against their use. However, in the real world many people

---

* Transparency Market Research, 2014.

prefer to consider the pros and cons of taking supplements, notwith-standing such risk.

In this second edition, I have added many new products and sifted through hundreds of scientific studies on sports supplements to cut through the hype and find out what works. The result is an inde-pendent evaluation of the most popular sports supplements. It will provide you with relevant and evidence-based advice so that, if you are considering taking supplements, then you will be able to make properly informed decisions.

Anita Bean
March 2015

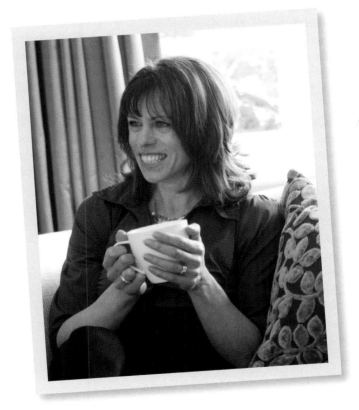

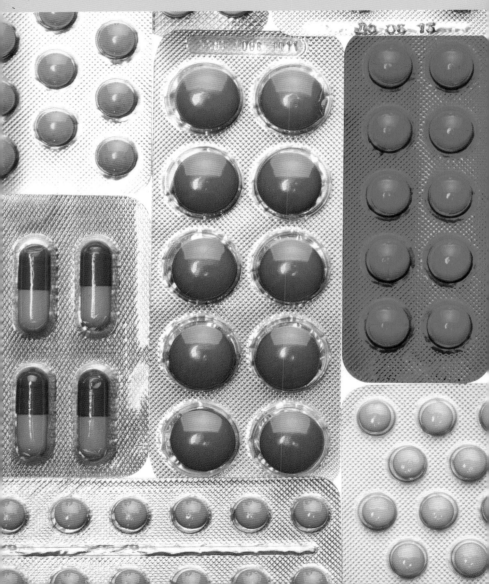

PART ONE

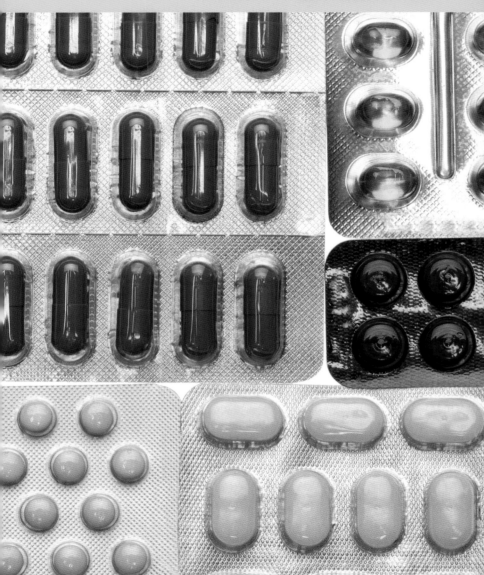

THE SCIENCE OF
SUPPLEMENTS

WHAT ARE SPORTS SUPPLEMENTS AND ERGOGENIC AIDS?

Sports supplements are a category of nutritional supplements whose purpose is to serve as an addition to the normal diet to improve general health and wellbeing or enhance sporting performance.

Supplements may include tablets, capsules, powders, drinks and bars, which claim to help with building muscle; increase endurance, weight gain or loss; improve suppleness; rehydrate; aid recovery or overcome a mineral deficiency.

Ergogenic aids are defined as any external influence created to enhance sport performance. They can include sports supplements as well as illegal drugs and methods.

The idea that certain substances or food ingredients enhance sports performance is certainly not new. In the ancient Greek Olympic Games 4000 years ago, athletes were reported to consume deer liver and lion heart to increase their speed, bravery and strength. Clearly, such practices were unfounded scientifically and based purely on belief, but they do underline the inherent desire in athletes to gain the competitive edge.

Nowadays athletes are faced with a bewildering choice of pills, potions, powders, drinks and bars promising greater stamina, increased strength, quicker recovery or less body fat. Some are supported by scientific evidence; many others are not. The question is how do you know if they are safe, effective and legal? Unfortunately, it's not easy. Unlike medicines, there's no systematic regulation of sports and other dietary supplements, or herbal remedies, so there's no way of knowing exactly what's in the product, nor any guarantee that a supplement works. Provided the supplement label lists the ingredients, manufacturers are free to make claims for enhanced performance, valid or not. What's more, advertising standards vary between different countries so some claims may be untrue or exaggerated. The trick is knowing which ones – if any – you should take, whether the product contains what's on the label and whether it lives up to its claims.

IOC CONSENSUS STATEMENT ON SPORTS NUTRITION (IOC, 2011)

The use of supplements does not compensate for poor food choices and an inadequate diet, but supplements that provide essential nutrients may be a short-term option when food intake or food choices are restricted due to travel or other factors. Vitamin D may be needed in supplemental form when sun exposure is inadequate. Of the many different dietary ergogenic aids available to athletes, a very small number may enhance performance for some athletes when used in accordance with current evidence under the guidance of a well-informed professional. Athletes contemplating the use of supplements and sports foods should consider their efficacy, their cost, the risk to health and performance and the potential for a positive doping test. Supplement use in young athletes should be discouraged and the focus should be on consuming a nutrient-rich, well-chosen diet to allow for growth while maintaining a healthy body composition.

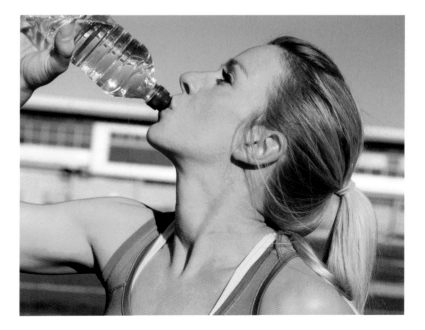

HOW WIDESPREAD IS THE USE OF SPORTS SUPPLEMENTS?

Many athletes believe supplements are an essential component for sports success and it has been estimated that the majority of elite athletes are using some form of performance-enhancing agent. A Canadian study of 440 elite male and female athletes found that 87 per cent used supplements regularly (Lun *et al*, 2012), while another Canadian study revealed that 98 per cent of young athletes aged 11–25 years used supplements either regularly or intermittently (Wiens *et al*, 2014). The most popular varieties are multivitamins, followed by carbohydrate/energy supplements, protein supplements, creatine and caffeine. Ephedrine, glutamine and HMB are also popular among strength athletes.

ARE SPORTS SUPPLEMENTS NECESSARY FOR MAXIMUM PERFORMANCE?

With the vast array of products available, it's tempting to think that sports supplements are essential for sporting success. However, this simply isn't true. Proper nutrition and training together with adequate rest are far more important when it comes to physical performance. Sports supplements cannot compensate for an unhealthy diet, inconsistent training, or inadequate rest.

Before you consider taking any supplement, make sure your diet, training and sleep are optimised. Think of these components as the base of a pyramid, providing a solid foundation of health. On top of this you can build nutrient timing and on top of that you can add sports supplements (see Fig 1). In other words, supplements are just the tip of the pyramid, or the icing on the cake. Taking supplements without first having a solid nutrition plan is like putting the cart before the horse. Only once you have the first three levels firmly in place can you begin to consider supplementation.

It's a good idea to consult an accredited sports dietitian or a registered nutritionist with expertise in sports nutrition, if you have any concerns about any supplements (see 'Resources', page 151). They will help you assess the associated risks and make informed decisions about the products. Do not rely on information provided by supplement manufacturers or advice given by unqualified individuals.

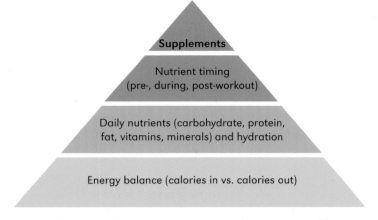

Figure 1: The nutrition and supplement pyramid

RISKS VS. BENEFITS

Sports supplements do not require UK Department of Health (DH) or US Food and Drug Administration (FDA) approval before they come on the market so there's no guarantee that a supplement lives up to its claims. While the regulatory organisations expect manufacturers to avoid making untruthful claims, these regulations are not well policed and supplements can be marketed with very little control over the claims they make.

However, supplement manufacturers do have to follow the DH's/FDA's current good manufacturing practices to ensure quality and safety of their product. The problem is that most health risks of supplements are discovered after the product is released into the marketplace, so the regulatory organisations can only remove a product from the market once it has caused a medical problem – and this is often a difficult and lengthy process. Supplements that are removed from the market are usually linked to a reported serious health risk or death.

Quality control and production standards vary considerably. While some companies follow good manufacturing practices, others do not, which means there is the risk that supplements could be contaminated with banned substances. This is known to be the case as many athletes have been tested positive through the use of supplements. According to the World Anti-Doping Agency: 'a significant number of positive tests have been attributed to the misuse of supplements and taking a poorly labeled dietary supplement is not an adequate defense in a doping hearing'.

Finally, it's worth knowing that the use of the terms 'herbal' and 'natural' on a product label is just a marketing technique – it does not necessarily mean that it is safe.

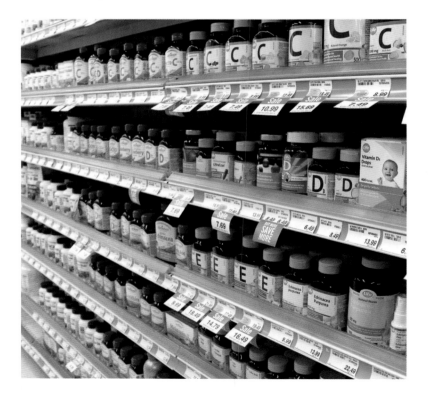

What are the risks with taking supplements?

If you participate in drug-tested sports you need to be extra vigilant with sports supplements as there is a significant risk of inadvertent doping. It is all too easy for supplements to become contaminated which could lead to a failed drugs test. In some cases, illegal drugs have been disguised as sports supplements and caused athletes to test positive for banned substances, resulting in serious consequences. Examples of prohibited substances that may be in dietary supplements are:

- Dehydroepiandrosterone (DHEA)
- Androstenedione/diol (and variations including '19' and 'nor')
- Ma huang
- Ephedrine
- Amphetamines

You should also be aware that some supplement ingredients (and medications) that are perfectly legal in Europe and the US may be prohibited by the World Anti-Doping Agency (WADA) for use in sport. For example, DHEA, a precursor for testosterone synthesis used for anti-ageing benefits, and sildenafil (Viagra), used for another type of performance enhancement, are two examples of substances that are perfectly legal for the market, but banned for athletes.

How widespread is contamination?

Studies have found that supplements are frequently contaminated with banned substances whether inadvertently or through poor manufacturing and/or inaccurate labelling of products. In a 2004 investigation conducted by the International Olympic Committee, of 634 supplements tested from 13 different countries, 94 supplements (15 per cent) contained prohibited substances that were not listed on the label (Geyer, 2004). Another 10 per cent showed possible presence of steroids. That means that one out of every four supplements contained prohibited substances. Products that tested positive were from all over the world. Of the 37 samples tested from the UK 19 per cent were positive and 19 per cent from the US were also positive.

Things have not improved. An analysis of 58 supplements purchased through standard retail outlets in the US by HFL Sport in 2007 found that 25 per cent contained steroids and 11 per cent were contaminated with stimulants. In 2008 HFL undertook an analysis of 152 supplements purchased through standard retail outlets within the UK and found that over 10 per cent were contaminated with steroids and/or stimulants (Judkins, 2008).

A 2012 investigation by the Medicines and Healthcare Products Regulatory Agency (MHRA) found that 84 illegal products such as energy and muscle gain products contained dangerous ingredients such as steroids, stimulants and hormones (MHRA, 2012).

According to a 2013 survey by HFL Sport Science, 10 per cent of a sample of 114 supplements and weight loss products purchased in Europe were contaminated with steroids and/or stimulants at levels that could have resulted in positive findings for athletes (Russell *et al*, 2013). Some of the contaminated products even claimed to have been 'tested by an independent laboratory' or that they were 'doping free'.

These cases show how easy it is to become a victim of inadvertent doping, not to mention the concomitant health risks.

ANTI-DOPING

The World Anti-Doping Agency (WADA) recommends extreme caution regarding supplement use as there is no guarantee that any supplement is free from prohibited substances. The World Anti-Doping Agency code contains the principle of 'strict liability'. That means that the athlete is strictly liable for any prohibited substances which are found in their bodies (urine or blood sample), so even if it turns out the banned substance was in the supplement but wasn't on the label, the athlete will face the same penalties as someone who deliberately took the banned substance. Ultimately, the responsibility lies with the athlete.

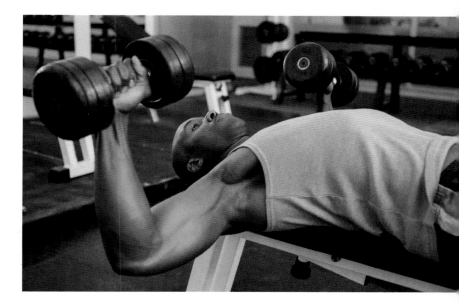

HOW CAN I BE SURE THAT A SUPPLEMENT IS LEGAL?

You can never be 100 per cent sure that any supplement is free from banned substances, even those claiming to be drug-free or safe for drug-tested athletes, for the following reasons:

- The WADA Prohibited List is not definitive – it does not specify every single substance that is prohibited, but instead identifies Classes of Prohibited Substances, such as anabolic agents and related substances, and Prohibited Methods only.
- Many analytical techniques have a finite limit of detection below which the technique will not be effective. This means that the presence of a prohibited substance in a supplement product below these detectable levels may still result in a positive drugs test.
- The sampling process for supplement testing is inherently inadequate for elite level sport as there will always be a large part of the product that is not analysed and it may be this part of the sample that contains the contaminant.

HOW CAN I MINIMISE THE RISK OF INADVERTENT DOPING?

Adhere to the regulations of your sport. Athletes who take dietary supplements bear full responsibility for everything they ingest. Whilst the risk of using a contaminated supplement will never be eliminated, you can minimise the risk of inadvertent doping by:

- Choosing reputable manufacturers who can justify their claims with scientific evidence, and have their products screened to minimise the risk of testing positive for a substance on the prohibited list. Contact the supplement company to investigate what they do to screen for contamination.
- Looking for voluntary certifications by companies such as Informed Sport (UK and US) or NSF Certified for Sport (US) on the label, indicating that the product has been independently tested for banned substances (such as anabolic agents, narcotics, stimulants, beta2-agonists, diuretics). Informed Sport and NSF are quality assurance schemes designed to minimise the risk of inadvertent doping. Their testing methods are accepted as the gold standard. However, it's only a voluntary scheme – manufacturers are not legally obliged to test their products – and, to date, only a relatively small number of products carry the logo due to the high costs involved. If you're an elite athlete bound by WADA and choose to take supplements, it's safer to use these products, even if you or your team receives sponsorship from another supplement company. You'll find all registered products listed on the companies' websites: www.informed-sport.com and www.nsfsport.com.
- Choosing pharmaceutical-grade products. This may reduce – although not eliminate – the risk of inadvertently taking a contaminated or poorly labelled product.
- Avoiding purchasing supplements from a manufacturer who also produces supplements that contain banned substances, such as dehydroepiandrosterone (DHEA), because they are particularly prone to cross-contamination.

- Only buying products that list all their ingredients and their quantities, not proprietary blends, which don't tell you exactly what's in them.

However, it's important to realise that even when using certified products, you are still risking a positive drug test. Any product can be contaminated since there is nothing in place to prevent this.

WHY ARE CERTIFIED SUPPLEMENTS SAFER?

- They are less likely to contain banned substances – Anti-doping lab, LGC (Informed Sport) tests for 146 substances; NSF test for 170 substances that appear on the WADA Prohibited List.
- What's on the label is in the product and nothing else.
- They contain no undeclared ingredients or unsafe levels of contaminants.

UK SPORT POSITION ON SPORTS SUPPLEMENTS

UK athletes are advised to be extremely cautious about the use of any supplements. No guarantees can be given that any particular supplement, including vitamins and minerals, ergogenic aids, and herbal remedies, is free from prohibited substances as these products are not licensed and are not subject to the same strict manufacturing and labelling requirements as licensed medicines. Antidoping rules are based on the principle of strict liability and therefore supplements are taken at an athlete's risk and personal responsibility.

Issued in 2003 by UK Sport, the British Olympic Association (BOA), the British Paralympic Association (BPA), National Sports Medicine Institute (NSMI), and the Home County Sports Councils (HCSC).

THE NATIONAL COLLEGIATE ATHLETIC ASSOCIATION (NCAA) POSITION ON SPORTS SUPPLEMENTS

It is your responsibility to check with the appropriate or designated athletics staff before using any substance. The NCAA bans the following classes of drugs:

- Stimulants
- Anabolic Agents
- Alcohol and Beta Blockers (banned for rifle only)
- Diuretics and Other Masking Agents
- Street Drugs
- Peptide Hormones and Analogues
- Anti-estrogens
- Beta2-Agonists

Note: Any substance chemically related to these classes is also banned.

The institution and the student-athlete shall be held accountable for all drugs within the banned drug class regardless of whether they have been specifically identified.

N.B. The NCAA is the governing body for US collegiate student-athletes at member institutions. The NCAA guidelines regulate what can and cannot be provided to a student-athlete in accordance with the Restrictions By-Laws through the 'permissible' and 'non-permissible' lists. Professional sport organisations are responsible for their own by-laws and sanctions regarding banned substances.

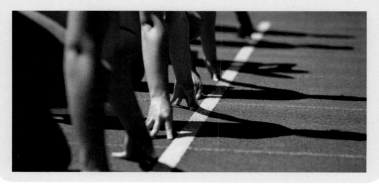

HOW TO EVALUATE SPORTS SUPPLEMENTS

- Don't be taken in by supplements that promise dramatic results. If the manufacturer's claims sound too good to be true, then they probably are.
- Be sceptical of adverts that contain lots of technical jargon or unnecessary graphs. If the information isn't clear and factual, leave the supplement well alone.
- Be wary of glossy adverts that rely on astonishing 'before' and 'after' photos rather than scientifically sound evidence for the supplement.
- Ask the manufacturer for evidence and studies that support the supplement's claims. If the information isn't available, don't touch that supplement.
- Check that any evidence is unbiased. Ideally, studies should have been carried out at a university, not funded solely by the manufacturer, and published in a reputable scientific journal.
- Don't take a supplement that has been recommended only by word of mouth. Check out exactly what is in it and whether it works before you buy it. Ask an expert if you have any questions.
- Be wary of supplements that contain similar endings to a banned substance. For example, supplements ending in 'one' are likely to have a similar chemical structure to testosterone.

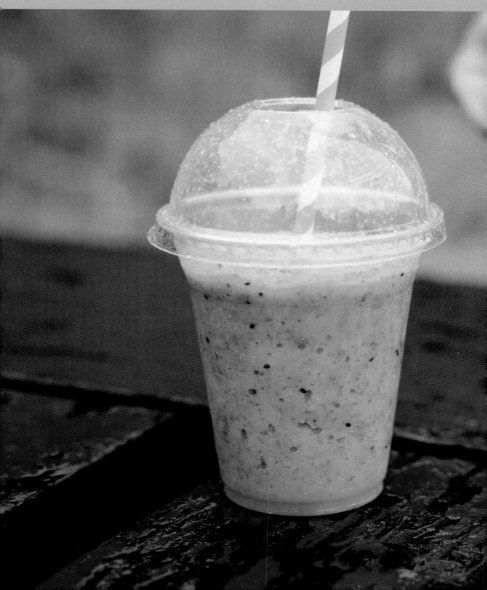

PART TWO

A-Z SUPPLEMENT GUIDE

ALL-IN-ONE SUPPLEMENTS

What are they?

All-in-one supplements contain a mixture of protein (usually in the form of whey, or a blend of whey and casein) and carbohydrate (sugar, maltodextrin or oats), along with other nutrients and ergogenic substances which may include vitamins, minerals, creatine, glutamine, HMB, beta-alanine, branched-chain amino acids and leucine. They are marketed primarily to bodybuilders for promoting muscle growth and recovery. Weight gain formulas are similar to all-in-one products, but usually contain more calories in the form of carbohydrates and fats to boost the calorie density.

How do they work?

All-in-one supplements provide a convenient way of obtaining several supplements in one product. The mechanisms of action of individual ingredients are explained in the respective sub-sections in this book.

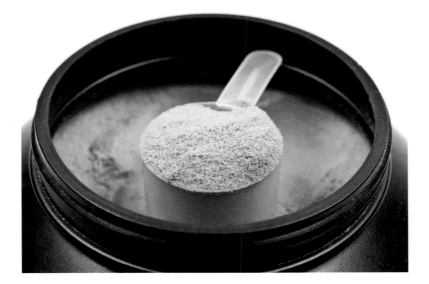

What is the evidence?

Although the effects of all-in-one products have not been directly assessed in studies, there is good evidence to support some of their key ingredients such as whey protein, creatine and beta-alanine.

Whey may help increase muscle synthesis following resistance training, although supplements are not necessarily superior to real food sources, such as milk (see 'whey protein', page 123). The optimal post-training dose is 15–25 g (Moore *et al*, 2009). One study found that athletes who consumed 20 g of whey supplement before and after resistance exercise had greater increases in muscle mass and muscle strength compared with those taking a placebo (Willoughby *et al*, 2007). However, consuming any high-quality protein source immediately after resistance training will also promote muscle repair and growth (Tipton *et al*, 2004).

Creatine is also a useful ingredient (see 'creatine', page 50). Hundreds of studies have shown that it can help increase strength, muscle mass, power and speed as well as enhance performance in high-intensity activities (Gualano *et al*, 2012). It has also been shown to enhance recovery after strenuous exercise.

Beta-alanine is a pH buffer that has been shown to improve performance in high-intensity events lasting between one and four minutes in both competitive and recreational athletes (see 'beta-alanine', page 33).

Some products contain glutamine, which manufacturers claim enhances immunity during intense training cycles. However, the evidence for any benefits on the immune system or on performance is fairly limited (see 'glutamine', page 72).

Many all-in-one products contain branched-chain amino acids (BCAA). However, there is little evidence to support the use of high doses (see 'branched-chain amino acids', page 38). Although BCAAs may help reduce muscle protein breakdown and promote muscle synthesis, you can obtain them from real food sources of protein as well as from whey protein.

Are there any side effects?
Side effects are unlikely.

Verdict
These types of supplements will not necessarily improve your performance, but are a convenient way to get your micro and macro nutrients for recovery. Most contain more than adequate amounts of high-quality protein (i.e. more than 20 g per serving) so they may be regarded as a good option when you are out and about or don't have the time to eat a post-exercise meal – although you should not regard them as substitutes for proper meals. Most are tailored to muscle building and may help take some of the guesswork out of supplementation for beginners.

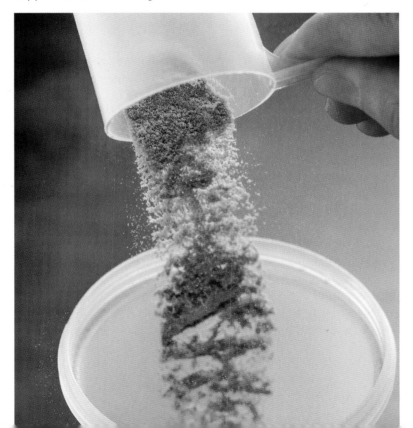

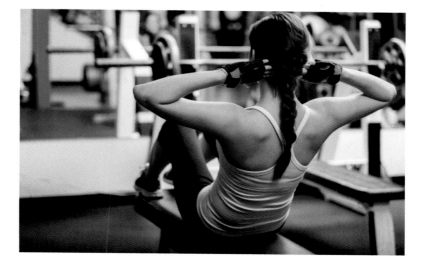

On the downside, they may not contain optimal amounts of nutrients such as creatine or beta-alanine, making them unsuitable for more experienced athletes and bodybuilders who require more tailored doses. On the other hand, the doses are probably effective for beginners and are unlikely to do any harm.

All-in-one supplements may also contain substances (e.g. glutamine) for which there is scant scientific proof, making them unnecessarily expensive. Check the amount of key ingredients on the label and ask yourself whether you really need all of them (i.e. is it worth the price?), and whether the doses are optimal for your sport and training programme. You may be better off consuming them individually so you can control the exact dose.

Finally, make sure you read the label very carefully! The list of ingredients is usually very long with many unfamiliar substances. In some products, these may include hard-to-spot potentially illegal substances that could cause you to test positive. If in doubt, opt for products that carry a voluntary certification logo on the label, such as Informed Sport or NSF Certified for Sport, indicating that the product has been independently tested for banned substances (see page 14).

ANTIOXIDANTS

What are they?

Antioxidant supplements may contain one or more of the following nutrients: beta-carotene, vitamin C, vitamin E, zinc, magnesium, copper, lycopene (a pigment found in tomatoes), selenium, co-enzyme Q10, catechins (found in green tea), methionine (an amino acid) and anthocyanidins 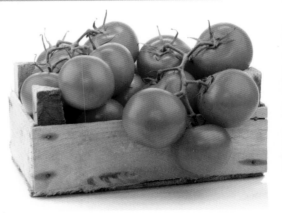 (pigments found in purple or red fruit).

How do they work?

The traditional theory, the so-called antioxidant-exercise hypothesis, suggests that intense exercise produces high levels of free radicals, or reactive oxygen species (ROS). These damage cell membranes and DNA and impair muscle function, hastening fatigue. The imbalance is sometimes called 'oxidative stress'. The idea behind antioxidant supplementation is to offset exercise-induced ROS damage and speed recovery.

What is the evidence?

Although previous studies have suggested supplementation may be beneficial, these are no longer considered valid due to small subject numbers and poor study design.

Newer studies suggest that antioxidant supplements either have no effect on performance or can actually decrease training efficiency and prevent adaptation of muscles to training – the very opposite of what athletes want (Nikolaidis *et al*, 2012). Although supplements reduce post-exercise oxidative stress, this isn't a good thing because oxidative stress is needed to stimulate muscle growth. In other words, oxidative stress and inflammation are desirable and are considered essential for training adaptations. ROS generated during intense exercise signal to the body that it needs to adapt to the stress of training by becoming stronger and more efficient. By prematurely quenching these ROS with high doses of antioxidant supplements, you could be preventing muscle adaptations.

Studies suggest that exercise itself increases the oxidative capacity of muscles by enhancing the action of antioxidant enzymes such as glutathione peroxidase and superoxide dismutase (Draeger *et al*, 2014). In other words, the body adapts to exercise by increasing its own antioxidant defences. Thus, taking supplements will provide no further benefit.

A review of more than 150 studies by Australian researchers concluded that there is insufficient evidence that antioxidant supplements improve performance (Peternelj and Coombes, 2011).

A double blind randomised controlled trial found that vitamin C (1000 mg) and E (235 mg) supplements blunted the endurance training-induced increase of mitochondrial proteins, which is important for improving muscular endurance (Paulsen *et al*, 2013). There was no difference in aerobic capacity (VO_2max) or performance between those taking supplements or a placebo. The researchers concluded that vitamins C and E hampered cellular adaptations in the muscles and therefore provided no performance benefit.

In another study, cyclists taking antioxidant supplements experienced no performance benefit during 12 weeks of strenuous endurance training compared with those taking a placebo (Yfanti *et al*, 2010). Similarly, another study found that vitamin C and vitamin E supplementation had no effect on muscle performance or recovery following four weeks of eccentric training (Theodorou *et al*, 2011). In another, footballers who took an antioxidant supplement experienced no increase in aerobic capacity (VO_2max) after six weeks of training, while those taking a placebo did (Skaug *et al*, 2014). In other words, supplementation with antioxidants appears to reduce rather than improve the benefits of training.

Are there any side effects?

Antioxidant supplementation may delay recovery and even result in reduced performance. A systematic review of 78 randomised clinical trials concluded that high dose antioxidant supplementation does not reduce the risk of cardiovascular disease and may, in fact, be harmful (Bjelakovic *et al*, 2012).

Verdict

There is no benefit to be gained from taking high dose antioxidant supplements. Instead of improving performance or promoting recovery, supplements may actually hamper it by disrupting the mechanisms designed to deal with exercise-derived oxidative stress. The consensus statement by the American College of Sports Medicine cautions against the use of antioxidant supplements (ACSM, 2009).

Getting your vitamins and minerals through a varied and balanced diet remains the best approach to maintain an optimal antioxidant status. There's good evidence to suggest that a diet rich in foods that are naturally high in antioxidants is associated with better health outcomes. The following foods are particularly rich in antioxidants:

- Red, orange and green vegetables (e.g. carrots, peppers, broccoli, cabbage, spinach)
- Red and purple fruit (e.g. strawberries, blueberries, raspberries, cherries)
- Onions, garlic, leeks
- Citrus fruit
- Nuts and seeds
- Whole grains
- Tea (black, green)
- Nuts and seeds
- Oily fish, avocado, eggs.

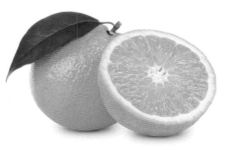

ARGININE

What is it?

L-arginine is a non-essential amino acid made naturally in the body. It is usually sold as arginine alpha-ketoglutarate (A-AKG) and arginine ketoisocaproate (A-KIC).

How does it work?

Arginine supplements are thought to improve performance by increasing nitric oxide (NO) production in the body. This is via a different metabolic pathway from inorganic nitrate found in beetroot/beet juice (see 'beetroot/beet juice', page 29). Nitric oxide is a gas that is involved in vasodilation, which is the process that increases blood flow to muscles, allowing better delivery of nutrients and oxygen. The idea behind supplementation is to increase the muscle 'pump' when lifting weights and promote recovery and muscle growth.

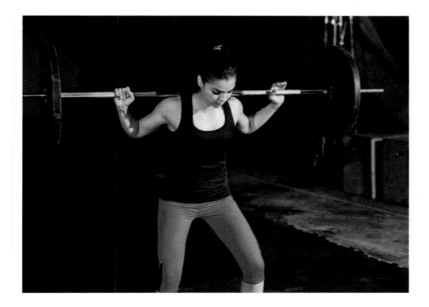

What is the evidence?

Little research supports these assertions directly. Most of the published studies suggest that arginine supplements have no effect on NO production nor intermittent anaerobic exercise performance in elite athletes (Liu *et al*, 2009). In one study, there was no difference in NO levels, blood flow or performance in athletes taking A-AKG supplements or a placebo (Willoughby *et al*, 2011).

However, an analysis of several studies concluded that supplements may produce a small benefit for beginners, but not for more highly trained athletes and not for females (Bescos *et al*, 2012).

Are there any side effects?

Side effects are unlikely from the doses recommended on the supplement label. Arginine supplements have been used safely with heart disease patients in doses of up to 20 g a day.

Verdict

Arginine is unlikely to benefit your performance – it does not increase NO levels to an appreciable extent. Other NO boosters, such as beetroot juice, are likely to be more effective (see 'beetroot/beet juice', page 29).

BEETROOT/BEET JUICE

What is it?

Beetroot/beet juice (and, of course, beetroot) is a rich source of nitrate. Nitrate is also found in other vegetables, such as spinach, rocket, celeriac, cabbage, endive, leeks and broccoli. To get the recommended amount of nitrate to enhance your performance you would need to eat at least 200 g (3–4 beetroots/beets) a day. Beetroot/beet juice is therefore a more accessible form of consumption.

How does it work?

The nitrates in beetroot/beet juice are converted in the body into nitric oxide (NO), a potent vasodilator (widens blood vessels) that helps increase blood flow and delivery of oxygen and nutrients to the muscles, thereby lowering the amount of oxygen needed by exercising muscles to sustain sub-maximal exercise (Bailey *et al*, 2009). Thus beetroot/beet juice may increase the muscles' efficiency and tolerance of high-intensity exercise and help increase endurance.

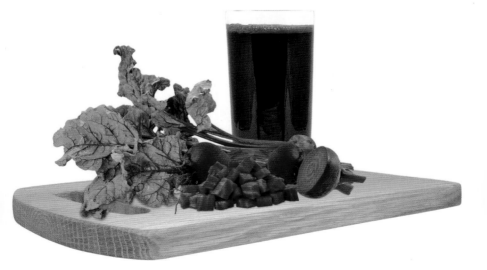

What is the evidence?

Since 2009, a number of studies with non-elite athletes have shown that nitrate in the form of beetroot/beet juice may help sustain higher levels of power for longer before fatigue sets in. In summary, it appears to reduce maximal oxygen uptake, improve exercise economy so you need less energy to do the same amount of work, and allows you to exercise longer.

Researchers at the University of Exeter found that drinking 500 ml of beetroot/beet juice a day for a week enabled volunteers to run 15 per cent longer before experiencing fatigue (Lansley *et al*, 2011a). These findings were correlated with the higher levels of nitrite measured in the blood, which reduced muscle uptake of oxygen and made them more fuel-efficient.

A further study by the same researchers found that cyclists given 500 ml beetroot/beet juice 2½ hours before a time trial race

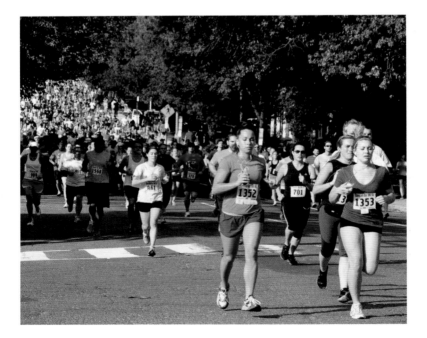

improved their performance by 2.8 per cent in a 4 km race and 2.7 per cent in a 16.1 km race (Lansley *et al*, 2011b). University of Maastricht researchers found that 170 ml of beetroot/beet juice concentrate over six days improved 10 km time trial performance (by 12 seconds) and power output in cyclists (Cermak *et al*, 2012).

One study found that whole beetroot/beet works equally well. Athletes who consumed 200 g cooked beetroot/beet an hour before exercise were able to run faster in the latter stages of a 5 km run (Murphy *et al*, 2012).

A review of 17 studies by UK and Australian researchers concluded that nitrate either in the form of beetroot/beet juice or sodium nitrate significantly improved endurance, as measured by time to exhaustion (Hoon *et al*, 2013a). Although time to exhaustion isn't a direct measure of performance, this finding could translate into a 1–2 per cent reduction in race times.

It's important to note that the majority of studies showing a positive effect involved untrained or recreational athletes, not elite athletes. Whether beetroot/beet juice also benefits performance in elite athletes is unclear. For example, Australian researchers found that beetroot/beet juice supplementation did not improve performance in competitive cyclists (Lane *et al*, 2013). Even when combined with caffeine, beetroot/beet juice (2 x 70 ml shots) made no difference to their performance in a 60-minute simulated time trial. Another study with competitive cyclists found little difference in time trial performance following beetroot/beet juice supplementation in competitive cyclists (Hoon *et al*, 2013b). So, to date, beetroot/beet juice appears to be a more effective ergogenic aid for non-elite than elite athletes.

Are there any side effects?
Beetroot/beet juice may cause a harmless, temporary, pink colouration of urine and stools. It may also trigger 'digestive distress'.

There have been questions as to whether beetroot/beet juice could theoretically increase cancer risk (dietary nitrates can be converted to nitrite in the body and then go on to react with amino acids to produce carcinogenic compounds called nitrosamines). However, research has shown that these harmful effects are associated with nitrates and nitrites from processed meat, not from vegetables (Gilchrist *et al*, 2010; Hord *et al*, 2009). The European Safety Authority states that the benefits of vegetable and fruit consumption outweigh any perceived risk of developing cancer from the consumption of nitrate and nitrite in these foods.

Verdict

If you're a non-elite athlete, beetroot/beet juice may help to give you the edge during endurance exercise lasting between 4 minutes and 30 minutes, or during intense intermittent exercise and team sports. Whether the same benefits apply to the elite athlete is not known for certain.

The exact dose and timing is unclear, but most studies have used doses of 0.3–0.4 g (0.62 mg/kg body weight), equivalent to 500 ml beetroot/beet juice or 170 ml beetroot/beet juice concentrate or a single 70 ml concentrated 'shot' or 200 g cooked beetroot/beet (equivalent to 300 mg nitrate).

However, the most recent research from the University of Exeter, UK, suggests 600 mg nitrate may be optimal, equivalent to 2 x 70 ml concentrated beetroot/beet shots (Wylie *et al*, 2013). The researchers also found that NO levels peak 2–3 hours after consumption and then gradually fall over 12 hours, suggesting that the optimal timing could be around 2½ hours pre-exercise. There was no benefit gained by taking more than 600 mg nitrate or 2 shots. Alternatively, according to one study, you may prefer to 'nitrate load' for 3–7 days prior to a competition to ensure your blood levels of NO remain high (Cermak *et al*, 2012).

You should avoid using antibacterial mouthwash as this may inhibit the transformation of nitrate into NO. The nitrate in beetroot juice is converted into nitrite (the first stage in NO production) by bacteria in the salivary glands. If you use mouthwash, then you will remove these beneficial bacteria and block the most important step in this process, thus greatly reducing the benefits of beetroot/beet juice.

BETA-ALANINE

What is it?

Beta-alanine is an amino acid that is used to make carnosine (a dipeptide made from beta-alanine and histidine). Carnosine is an important pH buffer in the muscles – it buffers the acidity (hydrogen ions) produced during high-intensity exercise, thus allowing you to keep going longer and combat fatigue.

How does it work?

Beta-alanine supplementation increases carnosine concentration in the muscle (Harris *et al*, 2006; Sale *et al*, 2010). These increased levels of muscle carnosine increase buffering capacity, helping offset the build-up of lactic acid during high-intensity exercise, which in turn may enhance sprint and short-distance performance. Normally, a build-up of acidity results in fatigue.

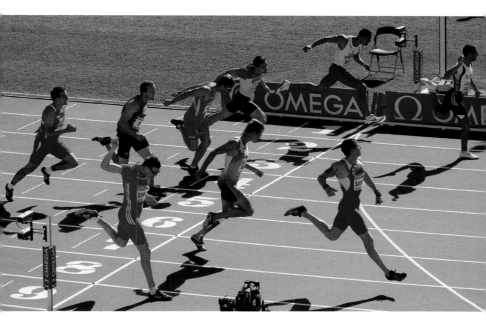

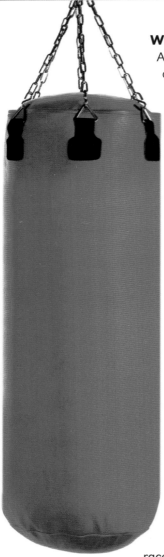

What is the evidence?

A systematic review of 19 randomised controlled (i.e. high-quality) studies concluded that beta-alanine supplementation leads to improved performance in short-duration high-intensity activities (Quesnele *et al*, 2014). Specifically, it may increase power output and anaerobic capacity, and decrease subjective feelings of fatigue and perceived exhaustion. According to an analysis of 15 studies, the average performance improvement is 2.85 per cent, equivalent to a 6 second improvement in an event lasting 4 minutes (Hobson *et al*, 2012).

Australian researchers found that runners who took beta-alanine supplements for 28 days achieved significantly faster 800 m race times compared with those who took a placebo (Ducker *et al*, 2013). The average times dropped from 2:25.7 to 2:22.1.

Another study measured significant improvements in power output and time trial performance in cyclists after four weeks of beta-alanine supplementation (Howe *et al*, 2013). Similarly, a study by Belgian researchers found that beta-alanine supplementation for eight weeks significantly enhanced sprint performance at the end of a simulated endurance cycle race (van Thienen *et al*, 2009).

Beta-alanine supplements significantly reduced fatigue in sprinters when performing a set of knee extensions (Derave *et al*, 2007). Another study at the College of New Jersey, USA found that beta-alanine resulted in increased training volume and reduced subjective feelings of fatigue in football players (Hoffman *et al*, 2008).

UK researchers found that four weeks of 6 g per day of beta-alanine (1.5 g, four times per day) increased the punch force of amateur boxers by 20 times, and punch frequency by four times, as compared to a placebo (Donovan *et al*, 2012).

Are there any side effects?
High doses may cause side effects such as flushing and paraesthesia (skin tingling). However, these symptoms are normally transient and can be prevented by using smaller doses or sustained-release formulations. The long-term effects of supplements are not known.

Verdict
Beta-alanine supplementation could be beneficial for activities that last between one and four minutes or involve repeated sprints or surges of power. However, the research to date has involved relatively small numbers of athletes, so opinions may change as further research is carried out.

Typical doses used in studies are 3.2–6.4 g/day for 6–10 weeks. However, the consensus appears to be that around 3 g (4 x 800 mg) per day for 6 weeks followed by a maintenance dose of 1.2 g/day gives optimal results (Stegan *et al*, 2014). The dose recommendations are not dependent on body weight.

As the performance benefits are based on raising muscle carnosine concentrations, it doesn't matter what time of day you take beta-alanine. You don't need to take it pre- or post-workout. The main thing is to take it consistently and, ideally, divided into several small doses (e.g. 4 x 800 mg). The clearance time of muscle carnosine is very slow, so once you've built up your muscle carnosine levels, they should stay elevated for a long period, dropping just 2 per cent every two weeks after you stop taking supplements.

BICARBONATE

What is it?
Sodium bicarbonate is a pH buffer that may help enhance performance in anaerobic and high-intensity exercise. It is a main ingredient of baking powder.

How does it work?
Supplements ('bicarbonate loading') will increase the pH of the blood and make it more alkaline. During high-intensity (anaerobic) exercise, hydrogen ions are produced, which gradually accumulate and result in fatigue. However, by raising the pH of the blood, hydrogen ions can pass more easily from the muscle cells to the blood, where they can be removed (buffered), which allows you to continue exercising at a high intensity for a little longer. It also means lactate is removed faster so you can recover more quickly.

What is the evidence?
Research has shown improvements in high-intensity events lasting 1–7 minutes. One meta-analysis found an improvement of 1.7 per cent for events lasting about one minute (Carr *et al*, 2011). A study with elite cyclists found that bicarbonate supplementation significantly

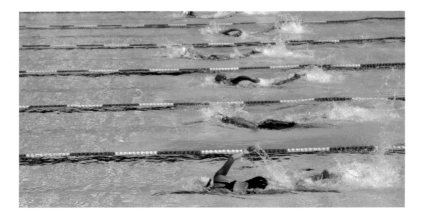

improved 4-minute cycling performance compared with a placebo (Driller *et al*, 2012).

However, not all studies have shown beneficial effects of bicarbonate. For example, an Australian study with eight swimmers found that bicarbonate loading did not result in faster times in 200 m freestyle (approximately two minutes' duration) compared with taking a placebo (Joyce *et al*, 2012). Another study with New Zealand rugby players found that bicarbonate loading produced no difference in performance in rugby-specific skills (Cameron *et al*, 2010). The discrepancies in findings may be explained by the fact that elite athletes already have enhanced muscle buffering capacity so stand to benefit less than recreational athletes from bicarbonate loading.

Are there any side effects?

Bicarbonate may cause gastrointestinal (GI) upset, nausea, stomach pain, diarrhoea and vomiting. These side effects could cancel out any performance advantage.

Verdict

You may benefit from bicarbonate if you are competing in high-intensity events lasting 1–7 minutes – e.g. sprint and middle-distance swimming, running and rowing events – or in events that involve multiple sprints – e.g. tennis, football, rugby. However, there is a high risk of side effects so you should try it first in training to find a protocol that works for you before using it in competition.

The most common dose for bicarbonate loading is 0.2–0.3 g/kg. This equates to 14–21 g for a 70 kg person. It should be consumed with at least 500 ml water 60–90 minutes before the start of exercise to minimise GI symptoms. Side effects may be reduced by taking the loading dose in several small doses and perhaps over an even longer period, along with a small carbohydrate-rich meal. Alternatively, if you will be competing in several events over a few days, you could try taking 0.5 g/kg/day over the course of 1–3 days, and then stop 12–24 hours before the event. Theoretically, the benefits will persist but with less risk of side effects.

BRANCHED-CHAIN AMINO ACIDS

What are they?
Branched-chain amino acids (BCAAs) comprise the three essential amino acids: valine, leucine and isoleucine. The term 'branched-chain' refers to their forked molecular structure. BCAAs make up one-third of muscle proteins. They can be found in any protein-rich food such as milk, eggs or meat.

How do they work?
Unlike other amino acids, BCAAs can be oxidised and used for muscle fuel. The theory behind supplementation is that BCAAs can help prevent the breakdown of muscle tissue during intense exercise.

What is the evidence?
Some data shows that BCAA supplementation before and after exercise may decrease exercise-induced muscle damage and promote muscle-protein synthesis (Shimomura *et al*, 2010; Jackman *et al*, 2010; MacLean *et al*, 1994). There is also some evidence that BCAA supplements may help preserve muscle in athletes who are dieting and, taken before resistance training, reduce delayed onset muscle soreness (Nosaka *et al*, 2006; Shimomura *et al*, 2010). On the other hand, if sufficient protein is being consumed then there appears to be little benefit in taking BCAA supplements.

What's more, there doesn't appear to be any significant benefit for endurance athletes. A study by researchers at Florida State University found that while BCAA supplementation before and during prolonged endurance exercise reduced muscle damage, similar benefits were obtained by consuming a sports (carbohydrate) drink (Greer *et al*, 2007). Similarly, a study of long distance runners found that supplements taken for seven days before a marathon did not improve performance, nor reduce muscle damage compared with a placebo (Areces *et al*, 2014). In other words, BCAAs do not appear to offer any performance advantage before or during endurance activities.

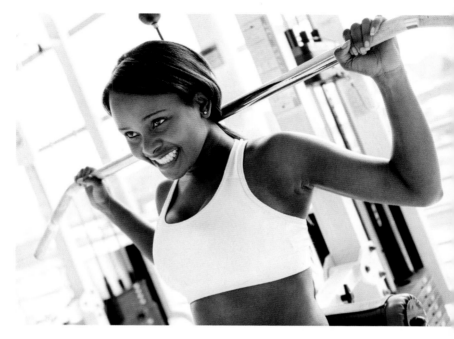

Are there any side effects?

BCAAs are relatively safe because they are normally found in protein in the diet. Excessive intake may reduce the absorption of other amino acids.

Verdict

There is little justification for taking BCAA supplements. A balanced diet with adequate protein should provide enough BCAAs. As long as you're getting enough dietary macronutrients – such as proteins, fat and carbohydrate – muscle will be spared. Theoretically, if you aren't getting sufficient protein in your diet or you're not consuming many food sources of BCAAs (e.g. dairy products), then supplements may help reduce muscle protein breakdown and promote muscle synthesis. However, it would make more sense to consume sufficient high-quality protein from food sources (1.2–1.8 g/kg) than to rely on supplements to get your amino acids, even if you are dieting.

CAFFEINE

What is it?

Caffeine is a drug rather than a nutrient. However, it is often considered a dietary supplement because it is found in many everyday foods and drinks such as coffee, black and green tea, cola, chocolate, energy drinks and gels (see Table 2.1).

TABLE 2.1: THE CAFFEINE CONTENT OF VARIOUS FOODS AND DRINKS

Drink/food source	Caffeine content mg per cup
Instant coffee	60 mg
Americano coffee (2 shots)	154 mg
Caffe Mocha (2 shots)	152 mg
Cappuccino (2 shots)	154 mg
Coffee (instant) (8 fl oz)	57 mg
Espresso (1 shot)	77 mg
Cafetière/filter coffee (8 fl oz)	145 mg
Latte (2 shots)	154 mg
Tea (black) (8 fl oz)	42 mg
Tea (green) (8 fl oz)	25 mg
Red Bull Energy Drink (8 fl oz)	80 mg
Coca Cola (12 fl oz)	34 mg
Coke zero (12 fl oz)	45 mg
Energy gel, 1 sachet	25 mg
Dark chocolate, 50 g/1.8 oz bar	40 mg
Milk chocolate (50 g/1.8 oz) bar	12 mg

How does it work?

Caffeine is a stimulant that acts on the central and peripheral nervous system. It works by increasing levels of ß-endorphins (hormone-like substances) in the brain. These endorphins affect mood state, reduce the perception of fatigue and pain, and create a sense of well-being.

Thus caffeine helps increase alertness, concentration and performance; and reduces fatigue. It can also help increase muscle fibre recruitment and thereby boost performance in anaerobic activities.

It was once believed that caffeine enhanced endurance performance by stimulating fat burning and 'sparing' the use of glycogen in the muscles. This is now known to be incorrect – any effect of caffeine on 'glycogen sparing' during sub-maximal exercise is short-lived and inconsistent – not all athletes respond in this way. Therefore, it is unlikely to explain the enhancement of exercise capacity and performance seen in many studies.

What is the evidence?

When taken ½–3 hours before exercise, caffeine has been shown to enhance performance in sprints, high-intensity activities lasting 4–5 minutes, intermittent activities such as team sports, and endurance activities (Burke, 2008; Goldstein *et al*, 2010). Benefits occur at modest levels – 1–3 mg caffeine/kg body weight, when taken before and/or during exercise. This is a lower dose than has been quoted in previous research (6–9 mg/kg).

Caffeine in pill form seems to be more effective than coffee. In one study, runners were able to exercise longer on a treadmill after consuming caffeine in pill form (with water) compared with consuming the same amount of caffeine in regular coffee (Graham *et al*, 1998).

An analysis by UK researchers of 40 studies on caffeine and performance concluded that it significantly improves endurance, on average by 12 per cent (Doherty and Smith, 2004). One study with swimmers showed a 23-second improvement in a 21-minute swim (MacIntosh and Wright, 1995). Researchers at RMIT University, Victoria, Australia found that caffeine improved performance by 4–6 seconds in competitive rowers during a 2000-metre row (Anderson *et al*, 2000).

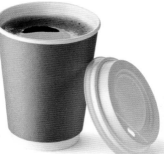

A study at the University of Saskatchewan found that consuming caffeine in amounts equivalent to 2 mg caffeine/kg of body weight one hour before exercise significantly increased bench press muscle endurance (Forbes *et al*, 2007). Another study with footballers found that consuming a caffeinated drink one hour before training and then at 15-minute intervals improved sprinting performance and reduced the perception of fatigue (Gant *et al*, 2010).

Caffeine also appears to benefit performance in team sports. Women soccer players who consumed 3 mg caffeine/kg of body weight in the form of an energy drink were able to run further and faster in a simulated match (Lara *et al*, 2014).

Are there any side effects?
The effect of caffeine on the body differs between individuals. Some people experience a performance benefit, some do not respond to it, while others experience side effects such as tremors, increased heart rate and headaches. These side effects are more common at higher doses, i.e. 6–9 mg caffeine/kg.

Other side effects caused by taking too large a dose include nausea, irritability, diarrhoea, insomnia, trembling and nervousness.

Verdict
There's good evidence that caffeine enhances performance for most types of endurance, power and strength activities. It does not enhance weight loss, but may delay fatigue and improve mental sharpness.

Although it is classed as a stimulant it is deemed legal in most drug-tested competitions. It was removed from the World Anti-Doping Agency's (WADA) banned substance list in January 2004. This change was based on the recognition that caffeine enhances performance at doses that are indistinguishable from everyday caffeine use, and that the previous practice of monitoring caffeine use via urinary caffeine concentrations is not reliable. It does, however, remain on the monitoring programme and may be added to the prohibited list again if it is found to be misused. However, it is banned by the National Collegiate Athletic Association (NCAA) in the US in high amounts (>15 ug/mL in the urine). This level would equate to about 500 mg caffeine taken pre-competition.

Performance benefits occur soon after consumption, so you may take caffeine 30–60 minutes before exercise, during your session (if you are exercising longer than an hour) or during the latter stages as fatigue begins to occur. It appears that relatively low doses (1–3 mg caffeine/kg) are just as effective as higher doses. This equates to 70–210 mg caffeine (equivalent to approximately two cups of coffee) for a 70 kg person, although it appears to be more potent when consumed in pill or capsule form than as coffee. You may prefer to take a caffeine pill or 'energy shots' if you want to get a precise dose. As individual responses vary, you should experiment during training – not during competition – to find the dose and protocol that suits you.

Sometimes athletes cut out caffeine from their diet for a few days or significantly reduce their intake prior to a competition. The idea is to reduce your tolerance so that when you reintroduce caffeine to your system, you'll get a greater response again. However, studies have found that there is no difference in the performance response to caffeine between non-users and users of caffeine, and that withdrawing athletes from caffeine does not increase the net improvement in performance achieved with caffeine supplementation.

DOES CAFFEINE DEHYDRATE YOU?

Although caffeine is a diuretic (i.e. promotes the production of urine), studies have shown that regular but moderate caffeine intake does not dehydrate the body as was once thought (Silva *et al*, 2013). Only if caffeine is taken in large doses – equivalent to more than 300 mg or three cups of coffee – or infrequently is it likely to have a noticeable diuretic effect. You can build up a tolerance to caffeine so its diuretic action becomes weakened if you consume it regularly. Taking caffeine during or after exercise does not dehydrate you either as adrenaline released during exercise blocks caffeine's effect on the kidneys (Goldstein *et al*, 2010).

CARNITINE

What is it?

Carnitine is a non-essential amino acid made in the liver from the amino acids lysine and methionine. It is essential for energy production and for fat metabolism. It can also be found in meat and dairy products. Most brands of supplements are sold as acetyl-L-carnitine, which is a better absorbed form of carnitine.

How does it work?

The main role of carnitine is to transport fatty acids into the mitochondria – the powerhouses of cells – where they are used for energy. The idea behind supplementation is that increased levels of carnitine may help the body burn more fat. Theoretically, this would be advantageous for weight loss as well as for endurance exercise. A greater reliance on fat for energy during exercise would help spare muscle glycogen and delay fatigue.

What's the evidence?

Despite the marketing hype, there is little scientific evidence to support these theories. While initial studies in the 1980s suggested a performance benefit, more recent studies have failed to show that supplements increase fat burning or improve endurance performance.

In one study, elite swimmers taking carnitine supplements for seven days did not perform significantly better than those taking a placebo during repeated 100 yard sprints (Trappe et al, 1994). Although supplementation raised blood levels of carnitine, it did not produce any performance benefit.

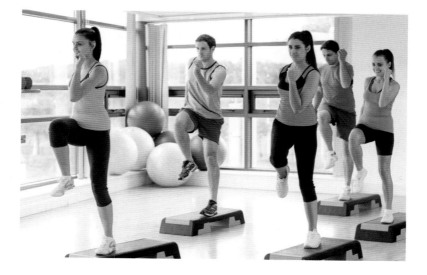

In another study, 14 days of carnitine supplementation failed to raise muscle carnitine levels or improve performance in a high-intensity sprint cycling test compared with a placebo (Barnett *et al*, 1994). A more recent study at the University of Memphis found that carnitine supplementation for eight weeks in conjunction with aerobic training did not boost muscle carnitine content nor benefit aerobic or anaerobic performance (Smith *et al*, 2008).

There's no evidence that carnitine promotes weight loss either. One Australian study with overweight women found that supplementation in conjunction with aerobic training for eight weeks did not result in greater weight loss than with a placebo (Villani *et al*, 2000).

Are there any side effects?
No side effects have been reported.

Verdict
As there is little evidence to support the claims made for acetyl-L-carnitine, it cannot be recommended as a performance-boosting or fat-loss supplement to athletes.

CASEIN

What is it?

Casein is a milk protein – it makes up 80 per cent of protein found in milk. It is available as calcium caseinate (a powder which can be mixed with milk or water to make a shake) but is also a major ingredient in protein supplements and all-in-one products.

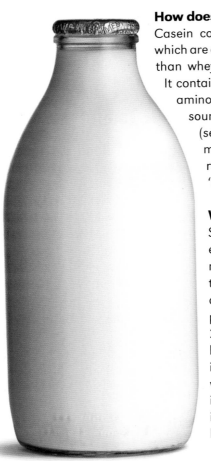

How does it work?

Casein comprises large protein molecules, which are digested and absorbed more slowly than whey (see 'Whey protein', page 123). It contains high levels of the nine essential amino acids. Casein is an especially rich source of the amino acid glutamine (see 'Glutamine', page 72). It digests more slowly than whey and for this reason is sometimes considered a 'slow-release' protein.

What's the evidence?

Studies have shown that consuming either a casein or whey supplement immediately after resistance training raises blood levels of amino acids and promotes muscle protein synthesis (Tipton *et al*, 2004). However, whey may be a better option than casein in the immediate post-exercise period as whey is absorbed quicker, but there is no evidence that either result in greater muscle growth over 24 hours (Tang *et al*, 2009).

In studies where athletes were

already consuming adequate amounts of protein in their diet, taking additional protein in the form of supplements before and after their workouts made no difference to muscle synthesis or strength (Weisgarber *et al*, 2012). However, as casein is a 'slow-acting' protein, it may be beneficial taken before sleep for promoting overnight recovery. A study at Maastrict University in the Netherlands found that protein synthesis was 22 per cent higher in resistance-trained males who consumed 40 g of protein in the form of a casein drink before sleep (Res *et al*, 2012). Casein produced a sustained rise in amino acids throughout the night and increased whole body protein synthesis compared with a placebo.

One study found that milk (which contains casein and whey) was superior to soy protein isolate in promoting muscle protein synthesis following exercise (Wilkinson *et al*, 2007). Another showed that athletes who consumed milk gained more muscle than those consuming soy protein drinks during a 12-week resistance training programme (Hartman *et al*, 2007).

Are there any side effects?

High intakes are unlikely to have any harmful effect in healthy people, but provide no advantage in terms of strength or muscle mass either.

Verdict

You may wish to add casein to your diet if you have particularly high protein needs (i.e. you weigh more than 85 kg/187 lbs and follow a strength training programme) or you cannot obtain sufficient protein from your diet. Because it digests more slowly and releases its amino acids at a prolonged rate, casein may be particularly beneficial before bedtime. Supplying the body with a slower release of amino acids at night appears to improve muscle recovery and promote growth.

On the other hand, you may prefer to drink milk, which contains whey and casein naturally and is cheaper. This is probably just as effective in promoting muscle synthesis after resistance training as supplements.

COLOSTRUM

What is it?

Colostrum supplements are derived from bovine colostrum, the milk produced in the first few days after the birth of a calf. Colostrum has a high concentration of immune and growth compounds, including insulin-like growth factor 1 (IGF-1), immunoglobulins (antibodies) and cytokines (immune cells) as well as various hormones and anti-microbial proteins.

How does it work?

It is claimed that bovine colostrum supplements enhance immunity during times of strenuous training, increase resistance to infection, and improve performance, recovery and body composition.

What is the evidence?

A number of studies have found a reduction in self-reported upper respiratory tract infections (URTI) following colostrum supplementation (Brinkworth and Buckley, 2003). One review of studies concluded that daily supplementation with bovine colostrum helps maintain intestinal barrier integrity, immune function and reduces the chances of

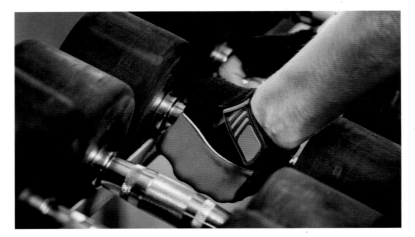

developing URTI symptoms (Davison, 2012). Another review of studies concluded that colostrum supplements may benefit performance and recovery during periods of high-intensity training (Shing *et al*, 2009).

The protective effect of colostrum is thought to be due to increased levels of bioactive constituents such as IGF-1, which enhances glucose and amino acid transport to cells and promotes muscle protein synthesis as well as increased levels of antibodies.

However, not all studies have found a positive effect (Crooks *et al*, 2006). For example, University of Queensland researchers measured an increase in immunoglobulins but no significant difference in incidence of upper respiratory infection among a group of cyclists during high-intensity training (Shing *et al*, 2007).

There is inconclusive evidence that colostrum supplements improve body composition, strength or power. One study at the University of South Australia suggests supplements improve anaerobic power after eight weeks (Brinkworth and Buckley, 2003). However, another study by the same researchers found that supplements had no effect on body composition after eight weeks of weight training (Brinkworth *et al*, 2004).

Are there any side effects?

There are no known side effects, but you should avoid colostrum supplements if you have a dairy allergy or intolerance.

Verdict

It is possible that supplements may help increase your immunity and speed recovery during periods of heavy training, but it is not certain whether they will reduce your risk of upper respiratory tract infection. Doses of 10–20 g a day for at least two weeks have been used in studies.

You should not take colostrum supplements if you participate in drug-tested sport. The World Anti-Doping Agency (WADA) recently recommended that athletes adopt a safe approach and avoid the supplement due to the naturally high quantities of IGF-1 contained in colostrum, a substance on WADA's prohibited list.

CREATINE

What is it?
Creatine is a protein that is made naturally in the body from three amino acids (arginine, glycine and methionine), but it is also found in meat and fish. As a supplement, creatine is most commonly taken as creatine monohydrate powder mixed with water, but other forms are also available.

How does it work?
The main way creatine supplements boost exercise performance is by increasing muscle stores of phosphocreatine (PC). This is an energy-rich compound (formed from phosphate and creatine) that fuels muscles during high-intensity activities, such as lifting weights or sprinting. Boosting PC levels with supplements should enable you to sustain all-out effort for longer than usual, and enable you to recover faster between exertions or exercise 'sets', resulting in greater strength and improved ability to do repeated sets.

Creatine may also buffer excess hydrogen ions during high-intensity exercise, allowing more lactic acid to be produced before fatigue sets in. It also helps promote muscle growth by drawing water into the cells, which increases muscle cell volume and acts as a signal for protein synthesis.

WHICH IS THE BEST FORM OF CREATINE?

Creatine monohydrate appears to be the most effective form of creatine. The only problem, though, is that the powder form is not very soluble and produces a chalky liquid when mixed with water. In practice, it is easier to mix into a milk or protein shake to avoid any chalky taste. Tablets and capsules may be a good alternative. Other forms such as citrate, phosphate, malate, pyruvate and serum are more expensive and less effective (Cooper *et al*, 2012).

What is the evidence?

Creatine monohydrate supplements have been well researched over the years and, on balance, have proven an effective aid for increasing strength and muscle mass, as well as enhancing performance in high-intensity activities (Gualano *et al*, 2012).

A review of 22 studies concluded that creatine supplementation increases maximum strength – i.e. 1 rep maximum – by an average of 8 per cent, as well as endurance strength – i.e. maximum reps at a sub-maximal load – by 14 per cent (Cooper *et al*, 2012; Rawson and Volek, 2003). Another review found that 70 per cent of creatine studies showed a positive effect on performance, and 30 per cent showed no effect (Kreider, 2003).

Creatine supplementation results in lean mass and total mass gains of typically 1–3 per cent lean body weight (approx. 0.8–3 kg) after a 5-day loading dose, compared with controls – although not all studies show positive results (Buford *et al*, 2007). The observed gains in weight are due partly to an increase in cell fluid volume (i.e. water weight) and partly to muscle synthesis.

One study found that creatine supplementation made no difference to body composition or strength in older males (aged 55–70) following a 12-week resistance training programme, compared with those taking a placebo (Cooke *et al*, 2014).

Are there any side effects?

The main side effect is weight gain. This is due partly to extra water in the muscle cells and partly to increased muscle tissue. While this is desirable for bodybuilders and people who work out with weights, it could be disadvantageous in sports where there is a critical ratio of body weight to speed (e.g. for runners) or in weight-category sports. Some people suffer from water retention, particularly during the loading phase.

As larger-than-normal amounts of creatine need to be processed by the kidneys, there is a theoretical long-term risk of kidney damage, but this has not been proven. One study found no evidence of impaired kidney function after 12 weeks of creatine supplementation

(Lugares *et al*, 2013). There have been anecdotal reports of muscle cramping during the loading phase, but this has not been proven to relate to creatine.

Verdict

There is an impressive amount of research supporting the benefits of creatine supplementation for power and strength athletes. If you train with weights, or do any sport that includes repeated bursts of high-intensity effort, such as sprints, jumps or throws, then taking creatine supplements may help increase your power, strength, muscle mass and performance. However, it is unlikely to benefit endurance performance.

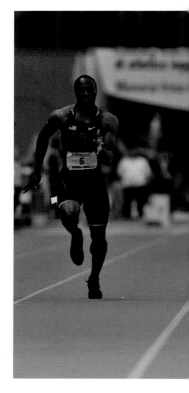

Be aware that creatine doesn't work for everyone – it is estimated that 20–30 per cent of people will not respond to creatine supplementation. The effectiveness of creatine depends on your diet (vegetarians may benefit more from supplements as they get none from dietary sources), fitness level, type of sport and age (older athletes are less likely to benefit).

The quickest way to increase your creatine stores is to use a 'loading protocol' of 0.3 g/kg of body weight for 5–7 days. For a 70 kg/154 lb person, this translates to 21 g/day. Take this amount in four equally divided doses through the day, e.g. 4 x 5 g. Alternatively, you can 'load' with a smaller dose of 2–3 g/day for 3–4 weeks to achieve optimal levels in your muscles. The end result is the same, whichever method you use. However, more isn't necessarily better! There is no advantage in taking more than 20 g/day, nor in loading for more than five days consecutively as your muscles have a maximum storage capacity. After your stores are loaded,

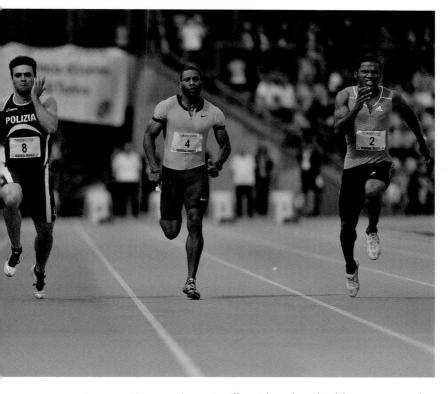

any extra creatine you ingest will not be absorbed by your muscles and will be excreted.

Following the loading phase your creatine stores can be maintained by taking 0.03 g/kg of body weight a day for no longer than one month. For a 70 kg/154 lb person, that's 2 g/day. The maintenance amount just needs to replace the amount of creatine degraded on a daily basis.

As creatine is stored in the muscles it can be taken at any time of day, before or after your workout. One study found no significant differences in muscle gains, body fat or muscle strength when body-builders took 5 g creatine either pre- or post-workout for 12 weeks (Antonio and Ciccone, 2013).

DEHYDROEPIANDROSTERONE (DHEA)

What is it?

DHEA is an androgenic hormone produced by the adrenal glands. Sometimes called 'the parent of all steroid hormones', it is converted in the body into several other hormones such as testosterone, oestrogen and progesterone. DHEA levels rise during puberty then peak around the age of 30, and then drop off dramatically in both men and women as they get older. By age 80 you produce only 5 per cent of the DHEA you produced at age 30. For this reason, it is often promoted as an 'anti-ageing' supplement. For athletes it is marketed for building muscle mass, increasing strength, decreasing body fat and increasing libido.

How does it work?

The theory behind DHEA supplements is that increasing blood levels of DHEA will also increase levels of testosterone, oestrogen and progesterone. For athletes, this would help increase lean muscle mass and libido as well as reduce body fat.

What is the evidence?

DHEA has been shown to increase testosterone levels, but only in males over 40 and post-menopausal women. There is little evidence that DHEA has a positive effect on body composition or sports performance. One study followed 87 men and 57 women aged 60 and older who had low DHEA levels (Nair et al, 2006). Although supplements did raise DHEA levels to normal, researchers found no significant changes in muscle strength or body composition.

A study of ten male bodybuilders (with an average age of 23), taking 50 mg of DHEA per day, did not report any improvements in strength and lean body mass when compared to the placebo group (Brown et al, 1999). In another study, supplementation with 100 mg DHEA failed to increase muscle mass, strength or testosterone levels in trained middle-aged men over a 12-week period (Wallace et al, 1999).

Are there any side effects?

Since DHEA is converted to testosterone, long-term use may cause potentially fatal liver cysts and liver cancer, increased risk of prostate and breast cancers, blood clotting, steroid-like side effects (increased facial hair, acne, mood swings), raised cholesterol and heart attacks. Long-term usage in women leads to the development of more masculine characteristics such as a deeper voice, excessive body hair and acne. In men, DHEA use can lead to gynecomastia (male breast development) due to increased oestrogen levels.

Verdict

DHEA cannot be recommended as a supplement and should not be taken by anyone competing in drug-tested sports. Its use is banned by all major sports organisations and it is currently on the World Anti-Doping Programme prohibited list (WADA, 2014). However, it can still be bought over the counter and from websites. You should be aware that samples may not be properly labelled – one study found big differences between the amounts of DHEA stated on the label and the amount actually present in the product (Parasrampuria et al, 1998). Some products claim to contain 'natural' DHEA precursors from wild yam. However, the body cannot convert these substances into DHEA. Only 44 per cent of samples contained what the label claimed, some contained only trace amounts.

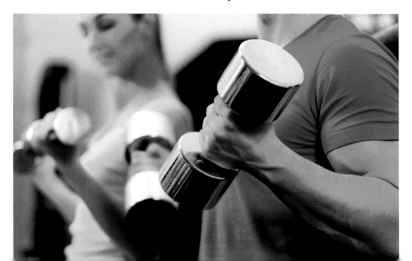

ECHINACEA

What is it?

Echinacea is a herbal supplement prepared from the stems, flowers, roots and leaves of the echinacea plant and is commonly used as a preventative for the common cold and flu.

How does it work?

Echinacea contains substances such as alkamides, caffeic acid and poly-saccharides that may help increase the number and activity of antibodies and other immune cells, thus helping boost immune function.

What is the evidence?

A Cochrane Review (a systematic review of primary research internationally recognised as the highest standard in evidence-based health care) of 24 double-blind studies concluded that preparations based on the aerial parts of echinacea purpurea might be effective for the early treatment of colds in adults, but results of studies are inconsistent (Karsch-Völk et al, 2014).

One study involving 755 healthy adults carried out by researchers from the Common Cold Centre at Cardiff University found that three daily doses of echinacea (specifically A. Vogel Bioforce) taken for four months reduced the duration and number of cold episodes by an average of 25 per cent compared with a placebo (Jawad et al, 2012).

However, another study found that echinacea pills were no more effective than a placebo for treating colds after symptoms start (Barrett et al, 2010).

One of the explanations for the discrepancy in results is that a variety of different echinacea preparations based on different species and parts of the plant have been used, making comparisons difficult. Generally pills based on root extracts are less effective than tinctures based on aerial parts of the plant.

Are there any side effects?
Echinacea appears to be safe at doses recommended by manufacturers.

Verdict
It may be worth taking echinacea as a preventative measure during periods of intense training when the body is more susceptible to infection. Under these circumstances, supplements may help to boost your immunity and reduce the frequency and duration of colds. Opt for tinctures containing the aerial parts of the plant rather than pills containing root extracts.

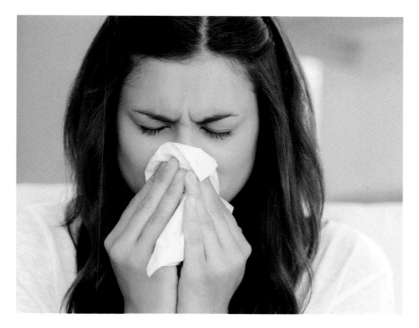

ENERGY BARS

What are they?

Energy bars consist mainly of sugar and maltodextrin; and provide around 250 calories and 25–35 g of carbohydrate/bar. Some may also have added vitamins and minerals, cereals or soy flour to boost the nutritional content.

How do they work?

Energy bars could provide a convenient way of consuming carbohydrate before, during or after intense exercise lasting more than one hour.

What's the evidence?

An Australian study compared an energy bar (plus water) with a sports drink during exercise; it was found that both boosted blood sugar levels and endurance equally (Mason *et al*, 1993).

In a study at the University of Texas, cyclists were given either a sports drink (containing 10 per cent carbohydrate), an energy bar

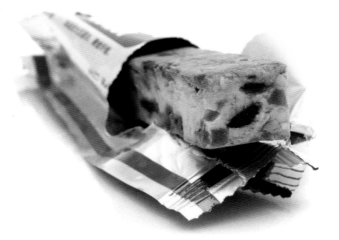

with water, or a placebo (Yaspelkis *et al*, 1993). Those who consumed some form of carbohydrate managed to keep going for 21 minutes 30 seconds longer before reaching exhaustion than those taking a placebo. The reason? The extra carbohydrate helped fuel the cyclists' muscles, reducing their dependency on glycogen. After three hours in the saddle, the cyclists sipping the sports drink or eating food had 35 per cent more glycogen than those who had consumed no carbohydrate.

Are there any side effects?
If you don't consume enough water, they may cause gastrointestinal discomfort. Some products may adhere to your teeth so ensure you rinse with water.

Verdict
Any form of high GI carbohydrate will help improve your endurance during high-intensity exercise lasting longer than one hour. Whether you consume carbohydrate in the form of an energy bar, drink or any other form during exercise is down to personal preference. The main benefit of energy bars is their convenience: they are easy to carry and eat! Make sure that you have your bar with enough water to replace the fluids lost in sweat as well as to digest the bar. They are an acquired taste and texture, and you may need to experiment with different flavours and brands.

Real food alternatives are bananas, granola bars or fig rolls. An Appalachian University study found that bananas were just as effective as sports drinks in increasing performance in a 75-km cycling time trial (Nieman *et al*, 2012). Trained cyclists consumed 0.2 g carbohydrate/kg of body weight every 15 minutes. On one occasion the carbohydrate was given in the form of a sports drink; on the other occasion they came in the form of bananas. It made no difference where the carbohydrate came from; the cyclists performed the same.

ENERGY GELS

What are they?
Energy gels come in small tear-off squeezable sachets and have a jelly-like texture. They consist of simple sugars (such as fructose and glucose) and maltodextrin (a carbohydrate derived from corn starch, consisting of 4–20 glucose units). They may also contain electrolytes (e.g. sodium and potassium) and caffeine. Most contain between 18 and 25 g of carbohydrate per sachet.

How do they work?
Gels provide a concentrated source of calories and carbohydrate and are designed to be consumed during high-intensity endurance exercise.

What's the evidence?
Studies show that energy gels are as effective as liquid carbohydrate (sports drinks) for fuelling muscles during endurance exercise (Pfeiffer *et al*, 2010). Consuming 30–60 g of carbohydrate per hour during prolonged exercise delays fatigue and improves endurance. This translates into one or two gels per hour. A 2007 study from

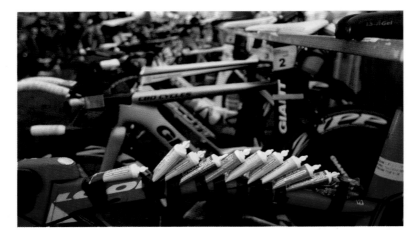

Napier University, Edinburgh, showed that gels have a similar effect on blood sugar levels and performance as sports drinks (Patterson and Gray, 2007). Soccer players who consumed an energy gel (with water) immediately before and during high-intensity interval training increased their endurance by 45 per cent compared with a placebo.

Are there any side effects?

If you don't drink enough water, they can cause stomach discomfort. They are very concentrated in sugars, so will drag water from your bloodstream into your stomach to dilute them, increasing the risk of dehydration.

Verdict

As with energy bars, any form of high-GI carbohydrate will help improve your endurance during high-intensity exercise lasting longer than one hour. If you have access to water (e.g. at race stations or water fountains), gels are a convenient alternative to sports drinks. They may help increase your stamina and performance during high-intensity endurance exercise lasting more than an hour. How much gel you need and how frequently you should take them depends on how hard and how long you're exercising. As a general rule, you'll benefit from 30–60 g sugar (one or two gels)/hour. Try taking a gel in the first 45–60 minutes of a race so you will benefit in the latter stages. Some athletes take a gel just before a race. Experiment with different doses and timings (e.g. half a gel every 20 or 30 minutes). Their caffeine content may also boost your performance by reducing the perception of effort and fatigue.

Always take gels with water to avoid gastrointestinal discomfort, but do not take with a sports drink otherwise you will have consumed too much carbohydrate. There are a huge variety of textures and flavours, so experimenting with different brands and flavours is very important for this category!

For real food alternatives you could try honey energy gels, which can be found in easy-to-carry pouches, or honey sticks, or real food such as bananas and dried fruit.

EPHEDRINE (MA HUANG)

What is it?
Ephedrine is a drug rather than a nutritional supplement. It is a stimulant substance derived from the ephedra or Ma Huang plant, often used as an ingredient in 'fat burners' or 'thermogenic' supplements. It is also used at low concentrations in cold and flu remedies (pseudoephedrine).

How does it work?
Ephedrine is a powerful central nervous system stimulant. It mimics the effects of adrenaline and norepinephrine, increasing the metabolic rate (by up to 5 per cent) and energy expenditure. It can also suppress the appetite. Athletes use it because it has a 'speed-like' effect, increasing alertness, motivation and performance. It also increases your heart rate and blood pressure as well as speeding up your metabolic rate and calorie burn. It is often combined with caffeine and aspirin or salicylates from the white willow tree as a 'fat burner' supplement – together they appear to boost each other's effects. Studies have shown that these supplements increase energy expenditure and help speed fat loss when taken with a low calorie diet. The problem is that they can also cause harmful side effects (see below).

What is the evidence?
Ephedrine is a proven stimulant. However, research studies generally show it has little effect on strength and endurance. This is probably because relatively low doses were used. What is more likely is that these products have a 'speed-like' effect; they make you feel more awake and alert, more motivated to train hard and more confident.

There is some evidence that ephedrine increases weight loss: partly due to an increase in thermogenesis (heat production), partly because it suppresses your appetite and partly because it makes you more active (Coffey *et al*, 2004).

When taken with caffeine, it is thought that ephedrine has a greater effect in terms of thermogenesis and weight loss. In one study, volunteers who took a combination of caffeine and ephedrine before sprinting achieved a better performance than those who took caffeine only, ephedrine only or a placebo (Bell *et al*, 2001).

Are there any side effects?

Up to 25 mg in one dose is considered safe in cold remedies; higher doses would be needed to produce a stimulant effect. The doses necessary to cause a fat-burning effect are quite high and are associated with a number of risky side effects including an increased and irregular heartbeat, a rise in blood pressure, insomnia, anxiety, nausea, irritability, dizziness, and other symptoms of nervousness (or being 'hyper'). More severe consequences of high doses such as heart attack, stroke and death have been reported in the medical press. Taking the ephedrine-caffeine-aspirin stack increases the chances of side effects even at low doses. In conclusion, the risks far outweigh potential benefits.

Verdict

Ephedrine cannot be recommended as an ergogenic aid. It is prohibited by WADA in drug-tested competitions (WADA, 2014). You should check the label of any cold remedies you may be taking to avoid the possibility of inadvertently testing positive.

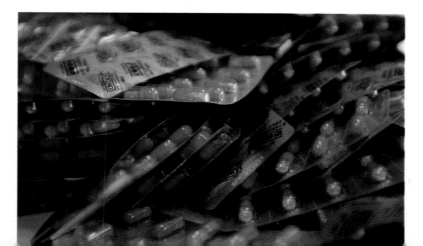

FAT BURNERS

What are they?

Certain fat-burning and weight loss supplements claim to mimic the effects of ephedrine, boosting metabolism and enhancing fat loss but without harmful side effects. The main ingredients in these products include citrus aurantium (synephrine or bitter orange extract); green tea extract and Coleus forskohlii extract (a herb, similar to mint).

How do they work?

Citrus aurantium is a weak stimulant, chemically similar to ephedrine and caffeine. It contains a compound called synephrine which, according to manufacturers, reduces appetite, increases the metabolic rate and promotes fat-burning.

The active constituents in green tea are a family of polyphenols called catechins (the main type is epigallocatechin gallate, or EGCG) and flavonols, which possess potent antioxidant activity.

Coleus forskohlii contains forskolin, which can be used to stimulate adenylyl cyclase activity, which will increase cAMP (cyclic adenosine

STIMULANTS

These include ephedrine, yohimbine, synephrine and methylhexaneamine (DMAA). They are banned substances, but frequently appear in over the counter and internet-bought products. These ingredients should only be available on prescription, but they may be found in unlicensed sports supplements, including 'fat-burners' or 'diet' pills. These claim to speed your metabolism, increase alertness, and shed body fat. But these stimulants are capable of causing significant side effects, such as increased and irregular heartbeat, raised blood pressure, kidney failure, seizures and heart complications. More severe consequences such as heart attack, stroke and death have been reported in the press. Several athletes have tested positive for DMAA and it has been linked to a number of fatalities.

monophosphate) levels in fat cells, which will in turn activate another enzyme (hormone sensitive lipase) to start breaking down fat stores.

What is the evidence?
Despite the hype, there is no sound scientific evidence to back up the weight loss claims of fat burners. The only ingredient that may have some value is green tea extract

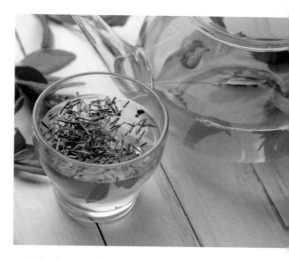

(see 'green tea extract', page 78). Research suggests that it may stimulate thermogenesis, increasing calorie expenditure, fat burning and weight loss (Venables *et al*, 2008; Dulloo *et al*, 1999). But there are no robust published trials showing that Coleus forskohlii extract promotes weight loss.

Are there any side effects?
While the herbal alternatives to ephedrine are generally safer, you may get side effects with high doses. Citrus aurantium can increase blood pressure as much, if not more, than ephedrine. High doses of forskolin may cause heart disturbances.

Verdict
The research on ephedrine-free fat burners is not robust and any fat-burning boost they provide would be relatively small or none. The doses used in some brands may be too small to provide a measurable effect. A careful calorie intake and exercise will produce better weight loss results in the long term. The only positive data is for green tea, but you would need to drink at least six cups daily (equivalent to 100–300 mg EGCG) to achieve a significant fat-burning effect.

FISH OIL/OMEGA-3 FATTY ACIDS

What is it?

Fish oil contains the two unsaturated fatty acids, eicosapentaenoic acid (EPA) and docosahexaenoic acid (DHA) derived from the tissues of oily, cold-water fish such as tuna, cod (liver) and salmon. The other main dietary omega-3 fatty acid is alpha-linolenic acid (ALA), which is found in rapeseed oil, walnuts, flaxseeds, chia seeds, walnut oil and flaxseed oil. ALA can be converted to EPA and DHA in the body, although with poor efficiency if the diet is high in omega-6s (found in vegetable oils such as sunflower and corn).

How do they work?

Omega-3 fatty acids are involved in a number of processes in the body, including the activation of 'locally acting hormones' known as eicosanoids, which control inflammation and immunity. They're also vital for the structure and fluidity of cell membranes. In addition, omega-3s are essential for growth, development, vision and the correct functioning of the brain and nervous system, with depletion associated with learning deficits. More recently, omega-3s have been linked with protection against depression, high blood pressure, heart disease, cancer, obesity and inflammation.

Theoretically, supplements are a good way of boosting omega-3 intake for people who do not eat oily fish regularly. Manufacturers claim they help reduce the risk of heart disease, cancer, type 2 diabetes, depression and degenerative diseases such as Parkinson's.

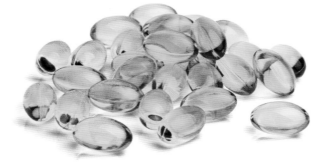

For athletes, supplementation may be a good way to help reduce inflammation in the body, including post-exercise muscle soreness; and improve muscle functioning, blood vessel elasticity and delivery of oxygen to muscles.

What is the evidence?

Fish oil supplementation in conjunction with exercise appears to have beneficial effects. For example, a study at the University of South Australia showed that overweight people who took fish oils while following an exercise programme lowered their blood fats and increased HDL cholesterol levels (Hill *et al*, 2007). They also lost more body fat compared with the control group who didn't take fish oils. In a 2010 study, scientists at Gettysburg College in Pennsylvania supplemented diets of healthy, active adults with either safflower oil or fish oil (Noreen *et al*, 2010). After six weeks, those taking the fish oil benefited from a significant increase in lean body mass and a reduction in fat mass.

One study found that omega-3s increased blood flow by up to 36 per cent during exercise (Walser *et al*, 2006). Another found that supplementation for 14 days reduced levels of inflammation after intense exercise (Phillips *et al*, 2003). Omega-3s also appear to play a key role in immune function. Researchers found 3 g fish oil supplementation for 60 days before a marathon prevented a drop in immune function induced by the race, although the researchers did not measure whether this led to a reduced incidence of colds or infection (Santos *et al*, 2013).

However, not all studies have produced positive results. In one, supplementation with 3.6 g fish oil/day for six weeks had no effect on delayed-onset muscle soreness compared with a placebo (Lenn *et al*, 2002). And, contrary to popular belief, omega-3 supplements appear to have no effect on cardiovascular disease risk. A systematic review and meta-analysis of 20 studies concluded that omega-3 supplementation is not associated with a lower risk of all-cause mortality, cardiac death, sudden death, myocardial infarction, or stroke (Rizos *et al*, 2012).

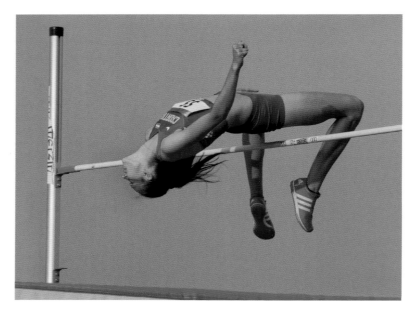

Are there any side effects?
Very high doses (more than 3 g/day) may increase the risk of internal bleeding. This is due to fish oil's ability to break down blood clots.

Verdict
Omega-3s appear to have a number of benefits for athletes, including improved blood flow and reduced inflammation, but it is unclear whether they can reduce post-exercise muscle soreness. If you don't eat oily fish regularly, two capsules of fish oil a day will provide approximately 500–600 mg of EPA and DHA, which is in line with population recommendations for heart disease risk reduction (Gebauer *et al*, 2006). The UK National Health Service recommends 450–900 mg of the long-chain EPA and DHA per day, which can also be met with two portions of oily fish per week. The American Heart Association recommends 1000 mg daily. However, based on the most recent meta-analyses, supplements are unlikely to prevent cardiovascular disease.

GINSENG

What is it?
Ginseng is the collective term for various extracts of the plant Aralia-ceae, the most important being the ginsenosides. The most common forms of ginseng include Korean (Panax ginseng) and Siberian (Eleu-therococcus senticosus).

How does it work?
Ginseng is known as an 'adaptogen' which means it helps the body cope better under stress. It has long been used to promote energy and vitality and, more recently, as a performance enhancer for athletes. Manufacturers claim that ginseng enables athletes to train more intensely, increases stamina and improves performance. However, the exact mechanism of its actions in the body is not known. One theory is that it influences the functioning of the adrenal glands and balances the levels of stress hormones such as cortisol. Another is that it acts on the hypothalamus of the brain and sympathetic nervous system to increase blood flow, oxygen delivery and use by muscle cells.

What is the evidence?
Unfortunately, there is a lack of scientific evidence to support ginseng's claims. Studies have failed to show that it increases oxygen uptake, athletic performance or endurance.

Are there any side effects?
High doses may cause high blood pressure and insomnia.

Verdict
As there is no good evidence to support the claims made for ginseng, it cannot be recommended as a sports supplement.

GLUCOSAMINE

What is it?

Glucosamine is found naturally in the body. It is an amino sugar, and a major component of cartilage, which serves as an important cushioning and shock-absorbing material for the joints. It is also one of the main substances in synovial fluid that lubricates and provides nutrients for joint structures. Supplements are made from crab, lobster and shrimp shells and sold in the form of capsules and tablets.

How does it work?

As the body ages, cartilage loses its elasticity and cushioning properties for joints, which may result in stiffness, immobility and pain. Sportspeople and regular exercisers sometimes suffer damaged cartilage as a result of years of repetitive motion and overuse of the joints. Glucosamine is thought to work by stimulating the cartilage cells to produce proteoglycans (building blocks) that repair joint structures. Thus supplements may help restore joint function and mobility.

What is the evidence?

Results of studies have been mixed. One review of studies concluded that glucosamine sulphate may be effective in delaying the progression and improving symptoms of knee osteoarthritis (Poolsup *et al*, 2005). However, a study of competitive male athletes recovering from acute knee injuries found that daily supplementation with 1500 mg glucosamine did not reduce pain or improve knee mobility (Ostojic *et al*, 2007).

In a large-scale US study (the Glucosamine/chondroitin Arthritis Intervention Trial, GAIT), researchers concluded that taking 500 mg of glucosamine three times a day; 400 mg of chondroitin three times daily; or a combination of glucosamine and chondroitin was no better than a placebo in relieving osteoarthritis pain after 24 months (Clegg *et al*, 2006). Similarly, a meta-analysis of ten large-scale randomised controlled trials (the 'gold standard' of studies) concluded that compared with a placebo, glucosamine, chondroitin, and their combination did not reduce joint pain or have an impact on narrowing of joint space (Wandel *et al*, 2010).

Are there any side effects?
Minor side effects may include stomach discomfort and intestinal gas.

Verdict
If you suffer from knee osteoarthritis, it may be worth trying glucosamine supplements, but do not expect miracles. Studies have used 500 mg three times a day. It may take three to eight weeks to produce noticeable results. Glucosamine sulphate has been shown to work more effectively when combined with chondroitin sulphate (a complex sugar that is found in cartilage).

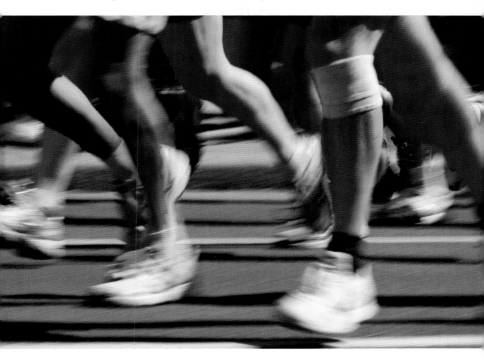

GLUTAMINE

What is it?
Glutamine is a non-essential amino acid found abundantly in the muscle cells and blood. It is found in high protein foods, such as meat, fish, milk and eggs. Glutamine can be taken as a powder mixed with water or added to a protein shake, or taken as capsules.

What does it do?
Glutamine is needed for cell growth as well as serving as a fuel for the immune system. The glutamine hypothesis suggests that blood levels of glutamine fall during periods of heavy training or stress, potentially weakening the immune system and putting you at risk of infection. Supplementation during intense training periods is thought to help offset the drop in glutamine, boost immunity, reduce the risk of overtraining syndrome and prevent upper respiratory tract infections. It has also been suggested that glutamine may help prevent protein breakdown during intense training.

What is the evidence?
There is little evidence to support the glutamine hypothesis. A review of studies concluded that while many athletes take glutamine supplements to protect against exercise-related impairment of the immune system, supplements do not prevent post-exercise changes in immune function or reduce the risk of infection (Gleeson, 2008).

One study found that there was no difference in plasma glutamine concentrations between elite swimmers who developed upper respiratory tract infections (URTI) and those who didn't during a four week period of intense training, suggesting that the incidence of URTI is not related to changes in plasma glutamine concentration (Mackinnon and Hooper, 1996).

To date, few studies have looked at the effects of glutamine supplements on sports performance. A review of studies concluded that there is little scientific evidence that glutamine can improve muscle mass, reduce body fat or improve performance (Phillips, 2007). One

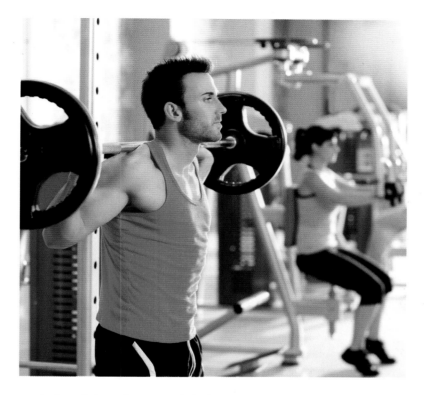

study found that glutamine failed to enhance high-intensity exercise performance in a group of ten male athletes (Haub *et al*, 1998). Similarly, Canadian researchers found glutamine produced no increase in strength or muscle mass over six weeks compared with a placebo (Candow *et al*, 2001).

Are there any side effects?

No side effects have been identified.

Verdict

Glutamine supplements are unlikely to be of substantial benefit in terms of preventing immune-suppression after exercise, improving body composition, strength or sports performance.

GLYCEROL

What is it?

Glycerol is a sweet colourless liquid found naturally in all fats in its glyceride form (it is the 'backbone' of triglycerides). It is used in food products, medicines and skincare products and is also a popular supplement with endurance athletes.

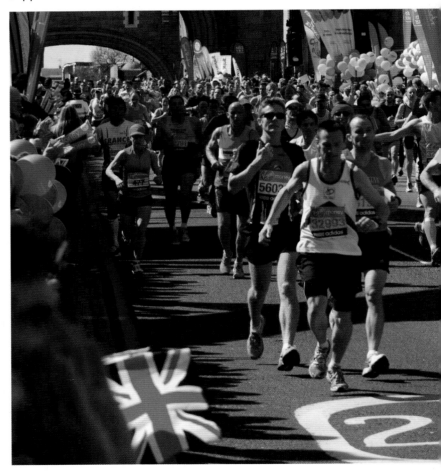

What does it do?

Glycerol is marketed as a 'hyper-hydration' agent. When taken with plentiful fluids before a prolonged endurance event (usually in the form of a drink), it increases hydration in the cells above normal levels. It does this by dragging water into both the extra-cellular and intra-cellular fluid and holding it there rather like a sponge. This results in an increase in total body water stores. This can be an

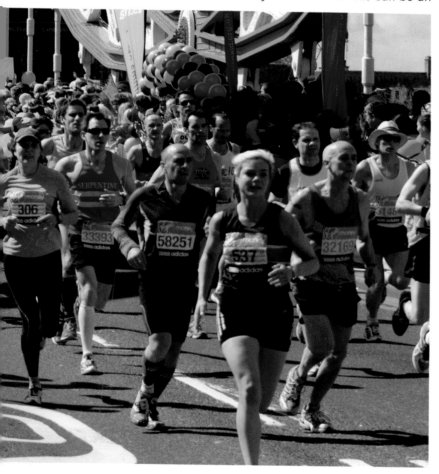

advantage during endurance activities because it allows the tissues to remain hydrated for longer. Thus it may help prevent fatigue associated with dehydration, and enhance endurance.

What is the evidence?

The results of studies have been mixed. Some studies have shown that drinks containing glycerol may improve endurance (time to exhaustion), time trial performance and power output (van Rosendal et al, 2009). For example, Australian researchers found that cyclists retained an extra 600 ml of fluid and improved performance in a time trial by 5 per cent following glycerol supplementation (Hitchins et al, 1999). Similarly, cyclists who consumed glycerol two hours before 90 minutes of steady state cycling experienced less cardiovascular strain and improved thermoregulation compared with a placebo drink (Anderson et al, 2001). However, other studies have found no performance benefits. For example, Canadian researchers found that a pre-exercise glycerol solution did not improve performance during two hours of cycling at 25 degrees centigrade compared with a placebo (Goulet et al, 2006).

More recent studies suggest that consuming a mixture of creatine and glycerol may be more effective. A University of Glasgow study found that male long-distance runners who consumed a creatine/glycerol drink twice daily for a week experienced less cardiovascular strain and better thermoregulation during a 30-minute run in hot conditions, but not in cool conditions (Beis et al, 2011). However, there was no difference in performance.

Are there any side effects?

A few side effects have been reported, including gastrointestinal upsets and headaches. If you wish to experiment with glycerol, follow the dilution directions on the label carefully and do not consume it undiluted.

Verdict

Glycerol is prohibited by the World Anti-Doping Programme (WADA,

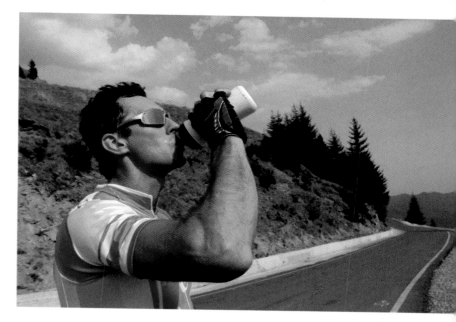

2014) so you should not use it if you compete in drug-tested sport. WADA considers it to be a 'plasma expander', thus making it a possible drug-masking agent. 'Plasma expanders' increase blood volume and circulation. Greater circulation to the muscles artificially improves athletic performance by increasing the delivery of nutrients to, and removal of waste from, muscles. In order for glycerol to reach such a plasma expanding effect, you would need to consume large amounts, far greater than found in normal amounts of food and drink. You will not test positive for consuming glycerol in foods and drinks, but you risk a positive test if you take glycerol supplements.

If you are not competing in a drug-tested sport, glycerol may help improve your performance in events where substantial dehydration is likely to be a problem, i.e. prolonged endurance activities in hot or humid conditions. Researchers recommend 1.2 g/kg body weight in 26 ml/kg body weight of fluid over a period of 60 minutes (van Rosendal *et al*, 2010).

GREEN TEA EXTRACT

What is it?

Green tea extract is a popular ingredient in weight loss and fat-burning or thermogenic supplements. The active compounds in green tea are a family of polyphenols (catechins) and flavanols, which are potent antioxidants, as well as caffeine. The main catechins include epicatechin (EC), epigallocatechin (EGC), epicatechin gallate (ECG) and epigallocatechin gallate (EGCG). A number of commercial green tea extracts are standardised to total polyphenol content and/or EGCG content.

How does it work?

Green tea extract has been shown to cause a mild increase in thermogenesis, i.e. calorie burning and fat oxidation. This is thought to be due partly to its caffeine content and partly to its catechins and flavanols content.

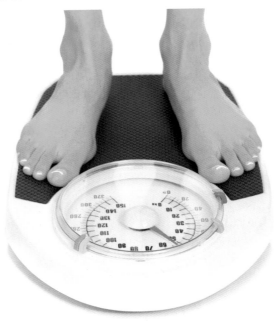

What is the evidence?

There is some evidence that green tea extract may be an effective weight loss supplement. In one study, volunteers were given either green tea extract, caffeine or a placebo (Dulloo *et al*, 1999). The green tea extract increased their daily calorie expenditure by 4 per cent while the caffeine supplement and placebo resulted in no increase in calorie burning.

More recently, a UK study found that people who consumed a green tea supplement 24 hours before exercise burned 17 per cent more fat during a 30-minute cycling test compared with taking a placebo (Venables *et al*, 2008). Thus green tea extract may have weight loss as well as performance benefits. If it can increase the proportion of fat and decrease the proportion of carbohydrate burned, it may be able to prolong endurance.

In a large US study, scientists found that people taking green tea supplements while exercising for three hours a week lost significantly more abdominal fat (7 per cent vs. 0.3 per cent) compared with the control group after 12 weeks (Maki *et al*, 2009).

However, not all studies have produced positive results. Danish researchers found that green tea extract did not significantly increase energy expenditure compared with caffeine or a placebo (Gregersen *et al*, 2009).

Are there any side effects?

Green tea is not associated with side effects, but high intakes may lead to restlessness, insomnia and headaches due to the caffeine content. If you are sensitive to caffeine check the ingredients on the supplement label.

Verdict

Green tea consumed either as a tea or as a supplement in doses of 125–500 mg per day may help you burn a few more calories in conjunction with an exercise programme. However, don't expect miracles – the increased calorie burn is small.

GUARANA

What is it?
Guarana comes from the seeds of a South American shrub. Guarana seeds contain twice the caffeine of coffee beans (3–7 per cent vs. 1–2 per cent). Guarana is marketed as a performance-enhancing stimulant as well as an ingredient in pre-workout supplements, energy drinks and weight loss products.

How does it work?
The active constituent of guarana is caffeine (the same caffeine found in coffee and tea) – typically guarana supplements contain 30–50 per cent caffeine. They also contain theobromine and theophylline. These substances are central nervous system stimulants and can increase the metabolic rate, increase alertness and reduce fatigue.

What is the evidence?
There have not been any studies on guarana and athletic performance. However, many studies have shown that caffeine can increase endurance and exercise performance (see 'caffeine', page 40). A review of studies suggested that any performance-enhancing benefits of guarana-containing energy drinks are attributable to their caffeine and sugar content (Ballard *et al*, 2010).

On its own, it is not a very effective fat burner although it may help suppress appetite. It is often sold combined with Ma Huang (ephedra) and aspirin. Such fat burning supplements claim to suppress appetite and increase daily energy expenditure, although the evidence is weak.

Some believe that the effects of guarana are less intense and longer-lasting than caffeine. Studies have not established this.

Are there any side effects?
Guarana may cause the same side effects as caffeine – anxiety, trembling, insomnia, headaches, high blood pressure and heart palpitations.

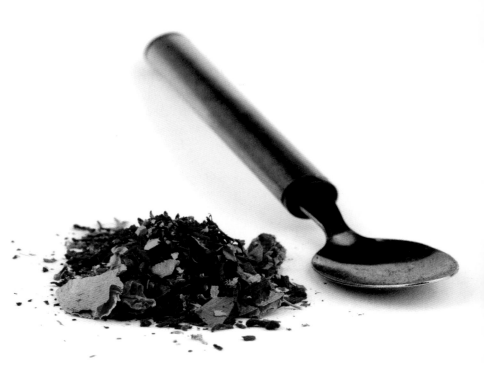

Verdict

Guarana may help increase endurance and exercise performance, due to its caffeine content. It's up to you whether you take caffeine in the form of coffee, caffeine-containing beverages or guarana – the only consideration is the caffeine concentration. Do not believe marketing claims that guarana is 'more natural' than other forms of caffeine or that it has no side effects. Guarana is not an effective weight loss supplement on its own.

HMB (BETA-HYDROXY BETA-METHYLBUTYRATE)

What is it?

HMB is the by-product of the body's normal breakdown of leucine, an essential amino acid. It also occurs naturally (albeit in small amounts) in citrus fruit, alfalfa and catfish. It is most commonly sold in tablet or powder form as calcium-HMB, which means the HMB molecule is bonded to a calcium molecule. However, it is also available as HMB free-acid (or HMB-FA), which is not bonded to calcium and claims to be more readily absorbed by the body.

How does it work?

HMB is a precursor to an important component of cell membranes that helps with growth and repair of muscle tissue. It is thought to work by reducing protein breakdown and increasing protein manufacture. Supplements may therefore enhance recovery after intense exercise and promote muscle strength and growth.

What is the evidence?

The evidence for HMB is divided. A number of studies suggest that HMB may have anti-catabolic effects, reducing muscle breakdown after resistance exercise, while others have found no beneficial effect.

A review of studies published by the International Society of Sports Nutrition concluded that HMB promotes recovery, reduces exercise-induced muscle breakdown and damage, promotes muscle repair, and increases muscle mass (Wilson *et al*, 2013).

But these benefits have not been found in all studies, particularly those involving more experienced athletes (Kreider *et al*, 2000). New Zealand researchers found that HMB supplements produced a small increase in strength in novice gym goers but not in more experienced lifters (Rowlands *et al*, 2009). One Australian study found that six weeks of HMB supplementation had no effect on the strength or muscle mass gains of well-conditioned athletes (Slater *et al*, 2001). Researchers at the University of Queensland in Australia found no

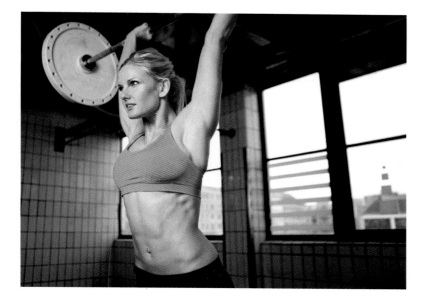

beneficial effect on reducing muscle damage or muscle soreness following resistance exercise (Paddon-Jones *et al*, 2001).

Are there any side effects?
No side effects have yet been found.

Verdict
HMB may provide muscle-building benefits for those who are new to lifting weights, but gains are likely to be fairly small compared with other dietary measures you can take. These include consuming enough calories (you should be in a slight positive calorie balance), carbohydrate, protein and fat. Establishing a good nutritional base and a consistent training programme should be your priority before considering supplementation with HMB. Studies have used doses of 1–2 g free acid form HMB 30–60 minutes prior to exercise (or 60–120 minutes prior to exercise if consuming calcium HMB) or 3 g (divided into 3 x 1 g doses)/day for two weeks. HMB is unlikely to be useful for more experienced athletes.

IRON

What is it?

Iron is a trace mineral, essential for the formation of haemoglobin, the oxygen-carrying pigment in red blood cells. It is also needed for a healthy immune system and preventing iron deficiency anaemia. Rich food sources of iron include meat and offal; wholegrain cereals, egg yolks, beans, lentils; green leafy vegetables, dried apricots, nuts, seeds, sardines and tuna.

How does it work?

Without enough iron in the blood the body cannot produce enough haemoglobin or red blood cells, which means less oxygen can be delivered to the muscles during exercise, leading to impaired muscle

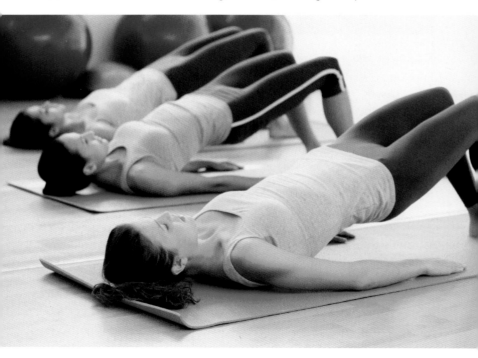

function and under-performance. The main symptom of non-anaemic iron deficiency is fatigue and a slight shortness of breath.

If untreated, iron deficiency can lead to iron-deficiency anaemia (characterised by low haemoglobin and a low red blood cell count); the main symptoms of which are fatigue, headaches, light-headedness and above-normal breathlessness during exercise. Iron supplements help to restore blood iron and haemoglobin levels back to normal, which in turn will increase oxygen delivery to the muscles and improve performance.

HOW COMMON IS IRON DEFICIENCY?

It is estimated that 30 per cent of female athletes, although not anaemic, have iron deficiency. This is termed 'non-anaemic iron deficiency', or 'latent iron deficiency'. Women in general are more susceptible than men to iron deficiency (due to menstruation) as are those athletes who avoid red meat (a readily absorbed source of iron) or eat very little (to maintain a low body weight) and perhaps do not compensate by eating other sources of iron.

What is the evidence?

There is evidence that iron deficiency, with or without anaemia, can impair muscle function and reduce performance (Lukaski, 2004). However, there is some controversy about what degree of deficiency supplementation benefits performance.

Many studies suggest that iron supplementation may be beneficial for athletes who are iron-deficient but do not have anaemia (Brownlie et al, 2004). It not only improves haemoglobin, serum ferritin levels and iron status, but also increases work capacity as evidenced by increasing oxygen uptake, reducing heart rate, and decreasing lactate concentration during exercise (Lukaski, 2004).

A review of 22 studies (encompassing 900 trained and untrained women) by researchers at the University of Melbourne found that iron supplementation improved maximal and submaximal exercise performance in women with or without anaemia (Pasricha et al,

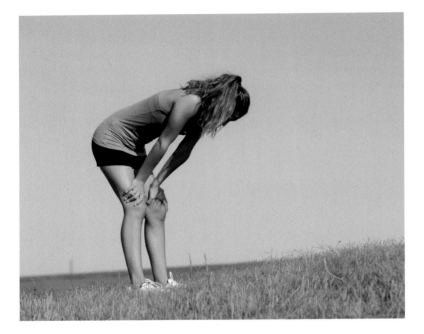

HOW IS IRON DEFICIENCY DIAGNOSED?

Iron deficiency is usually diagnosed by measuring ferritin (a protein in the blood that binds to iron), haemoglobin (the iron-containing protein in red blood cells that carries oxygen around the body), haematocrit (the volume percentage of red blood cells in the blood), iron, and total iron binding capacity (a measure of the blood's capacity to bind iron with the transporter protein, transferrin) in the blood. If you have iron deficiency, your iron is low, your total iron binding capacity is high (meaning there is lots of extra room to bind more iron), and your ferritin (a measure of your iron stores) is low. In incidences of anaemia, your haemoglobin and haematocrit, which are measures of your red blood cell count, are low. The average person will have normal ferritin levels of 12–300 nanograms per millilitre (ng/ml) for men and 12–150 ng/ml for women. It is thought that ferritin levels below 20 ng/ml can impair performance.

2014). The dose varied between studies, but significant improvements were seen both in women who were iron deficient, and those who were not, although the meta-analysis failed to distinguish between women who were deficient and those who were not. Heart rate decreased during submaximal exercise for the supplemented group, suggesting that oxygen transportation is more efficient with iron supplementation.

A US study found that six weeks of iron supplementation improved the iron status of iron-depleted female rowers as well as improved their time trial performance compared with a placebo (Dellavalle and Haas, 2013).

Are there any side effects?
Supplements at levels higher than 50–60 mg iron may cause constipation and stomach discomfort.

Verdict
If you have been diagnosed with iron deficiency, you will certainly benefit from iron supplementation. However, if you are not deficient then you shouldn't take supplements – they won't benefit your performance and may do more harm than good.

Iron deficiency is diagnosed with a blood test (see 'How is iron deficiency diagnosed?' on page 86). If you are iron deficient, your doctor will prescribe supplements. These may be taken in pill or liquid form, whichever suits you best. The usual recommended dose is 60 mg elemental iron taken in the form of iron sulphate for three months, although doses depend on gender, weight and iron level.

To maintain your iron levels, ensure you include iron-rich foods such as meat, liver, leafy green vegetables and nuts in your diet. Vitamin C (e.g. orange juice, strawberries, spinach) consumed at the same time boosts iron absorption.

ISOTONIC DRINKS – SEE 'SPORTS DRINKS' (PAGE 98)

LEUCINE

What is it?

Leucine is an essential amino acid, which simply means the body cannot produce it and we must get it from dietary sources. Leucine is the most abundant of the three branched-chain amino acids (BCAAs) in muscles (the other two are isoleucine and valine).

How does it work?

Leucine is an important trigger for protein synthesis. It acts as a signal to the muscle cells to make new muscle proteins, activating a compound called mTOR (mammalian target of rapamycin), and a molecular switch that turns on the machinery that manufactures muscle proteins.

What is the evidence?

Research suggests that leucine can stimulate protein synthesis (when consumed after exercise) and lessen protein breakdown (when consumed before exercise). In a study at the University of Maastricht, athletes who consumed a leucine/carbohydrate/protein drink after resistance training had less muscle protein breakdown and greater muscle protein synthesis than those who consumed a supplement without leucine (Koopman et al, 2005). Similarly, another study found that consuming a leucine-enriched protein drink during endurance exercise resulted in less muscle breakdown and greater muscle synthesis (Pasiakos et al, 2011). A study with canoeists found that six weeks of leucine supplementation improved endurance performance and upper body power (Crowe et al, 2006). However, there is no benefit in taking extra leucine if you consume protein (as food or drink) before or after exercise. Researchers found that consuming more than 1.8 g leucine does not produce any additional benefit (Pasiakos and McClung, 2011).

Are there any side effects?

There are no reported side effects.

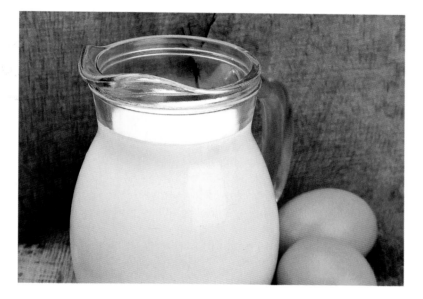

Verdict

Getting sufficient leucine is particularly important for those wanting to build strength and muscle mass. However, it isn't necessary to get leucine in the form of supplements. It is found widely in foods, the best sources being eggs, dairy products, meat, fish and poultry. It is also found in high concentrations in whey protein. You'll need around 2 g leucine to get maximum muscle-building benefits; that's the amount found in approximately 20 g of an animal protein source. Table 2.2 shows the amounts of various foods that you would need to consume to get 2 g leucine and 20 g protein.

TABLE 2.2: FOODS SUPPLYING 2 g LEUCINE AND 20 g PROTEIN

600 ml milk	85 g meat or poultry
85 g Cheddar cheese	100 g fish
450 g plain yoghurt	17 g whey powder
3 eggs	

MULTIVITAMINS

What are they?

Multivitamin and mineral supplements are available in pill, powder and liquid form.

How do they work?

Regular intense exercise places additional demands on your body, which means the requirement for many vitamins and minerals (micronutrients) is likely to be higher than the RDAs for the general population. Micronutrients play an important role in energy production, haemoglobin synthesis, bone health, immune function, and protecting the body against oxidative damage. They help with synthesis and repair of muscle tissue during recovery. As a result, greater intakes of micronutrients may be required to cover increased needs for building, repair, and maintenance of lean body mass in athletes. Failure to get enough micronutrients could leave you lacking in energy and susceptible to minor infections and illnesses.

What is the evidence?

Scientific evidence to support the use of multivitamins is lacking. Although supplementation may improve the nutritional status of an individual who consumes marginal amounts of nutrients and may enhance the physical performance of those athletes with overt

WHAT ARE RDAs?

The Recommended Daily Amounts (RDAs) listed on food and supplement labels are rough estimates of nutrient requirements designed to cover the needs of the majority (97-98 per cent) of healthy individuals in a particular stage and gender group. The amounts are designed to prevent deficiency symptoms, allow for a little storage, as well as covering differences in needs from one person to the next. They are not targets; rather they are guides to help you check that you are probably getting enough nutrients.

nutrient deficiencies, there is no scientific evidence to support the general use of vitamin and mineral supplements to improve athletic performance. According to the American College of Sports Medicine, the increased food intake of physically active individuals should provide the additional vitamins and minerals needed if a wide variety of foods is included in the diet (American College of Sports Medicine, 2009).

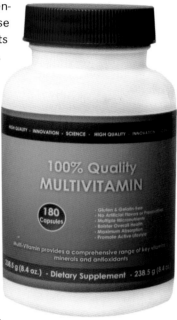

A comprehensive review of 26 studies concluded that for healthy people without nutritional deficiencies, there's little justification for taking multivitamins (Fortmann et al, 2013). Similarly, a large randomised clinical trial of male doctors aged 65 or older found no benefit from multivitamin supplementation for the risk for cancer, cardiovascular disease and dementia (Grodstein et al, 2013). However, the doses of vitamins were relatively low and the study participants were already 'well nourished'.

Are there any side effects?
Taking multivitamin supplements is generally harmless as amounts of nutrients are usually close to the RDAs. But you should check that they are all within safe upper levels. Tolerable upper intake levels (UL) are defined as the highest level of nutrient intake that is likely to pose no risk of adverse health effects for most individuals. While you would have to really overdo your vitamin and mineral intake to create serious toxicity issues, even moderate levels of 'mega dosing' can have adverse effects.

Verdict

If you are consuming a healthy diet that meets your calorie and macro-nutrient requirements, you probably won't benefit from multivitamin supplements. High doses will not enhance exercise performance or health. On the other hand, supplements providing approximately the RDA for most nutrients are unlikely to do any harm and may be regarded as useful insurance against deficient intakes.

Supplements are not a good substitute for food. Popping a pill can't erase the health effects of a poor diet and sedentary lifestyle. Go for real food first. Of course, more isn't better and it's important not to take more than the recommended dose. While supplements can help fill some of the gaps in a less than optimal diet, too much can be harmful.

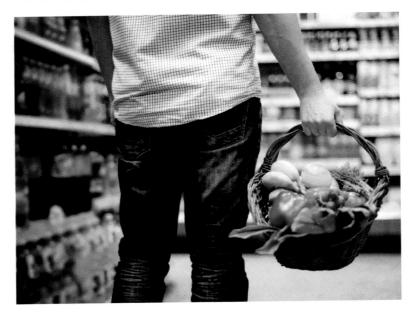

OMEGA-3 FATTY ACIDS - SEE 'FISH OIL' (PAGE 66)

PROBIOTICS

What are they?
Probiotics are the live microorganisms (bacteria) that live in the gut that are crucial for optimal intestinal health, digestion and immunity. They are found in yogurt and other cultured milk products as well as capsules, tablets and powders. The main commercially used species are Lactobacillus acidophilus, Bifidobacterium bifidum and L.casei immunitas cultures.

How do they work?
Probiotic supplements work by re-colonising the small intestine and crowding out disease-causing bacteria, thereby strengthening or restoring the balance to the intestinal flora. Thus, they may enhance the immune system and help protect against and reduce symptoms of gastrointestinal and upper respiratory tract infections (URTI). They may also improve intestinal tract health and increase the bioavailability of nutrients.

What's the evidence?
Hard training can put a significant strain on your immune system, increasing the risk of catching minor illnesses such as URTI. Studies show that various immune cell functions are impaired following prolonged intense training sessions. Probiotics have been shown to reduce the incidence of URTI in athletes during winter months, and may also reduce gastrointestinal distress often associated with longer bouts of training.

A study carried out by researchers at the Australian Institute of Sport found that probiotic supplementation can dramatically cut the risk and length of URTI in elite long distance runners (Cox *et al*, 2010). Those taking probiotic supplements experienced symptoms of URTI for 30 days during four months of intensive training compared with 72 days in the placebo group, and the severity of symptoms was less. This was attributed to higher levels of interferon (immune cells that fight viruses). In a follow up study with competitive cyclists, 11 weeks of probiotic supplementation reduced the severity and duration of lower respiratory illness by 30 per cent compared with a placebo (West *et al*, 2011). There was also a reduction in the severity of gastrointestinal symptoms, and athletes used cold and flu medication less frequently.

A review of randomised controlled trials (the gold standard for studies) concluded that probiotics are effective for preventing URTIs and reducing antibiotic use compared with a placebo (Hao *et al*, 2011).

Are there any side effects?
No significant adverse health effects have been reported.

Verdict
Taking a probiotic supplement during periods of heavy training or in the two weeks prior to a major competition may help to enhance your immune system and reduce the likelihood of getting a respiratory illness. Most studies have used doses of 1–10 billion bacteria/day.

Although probiotics are available in capsule form, ingesting them from 'live' yoghurt may be a cheaper alternative (a 125 g/4 oz serving contains around 4 billion bacteria), plus you benefit from additional nutrients such as calcium and protein, which plays an important role in muscle recovery and weight control.

PROHORMONES

What are they?
Prohormone supplements include DHEA, androstenedione (or andro for short) and norandrostenedione. They are marketed to bodybuilders and other athletes looking to increase strength and muscle mass.

How do they work?
Manufacturers claim the supplements will increase testosterone levels in the body and produce similar muscle-building effects to anabolic steroids, but without the side effects.

What is the evidence?
Current research does not support supplement manufacturers' claims. Studies show that andro supplements and DHEA have no significant testosterone-raising effects, and no effect on muscle mass or strength (Brown *et al*, 1999; King *et al*, 1999; Broeder *et al*, 2000; Powers, 2002).

In a double blind crossover study, researchers from McMaster University, Canada, found that androstenedione supplements failed to raise testosterone levels in the blood either at rest or following resistance training compared with a placebo (Ballantyne *et al*, 2000).

A study at Iowa State University found that eight weeks of supplementation with androstenedione, DHEA, saw palmetto, tribulus terrestris and chrysin combined with a weight training programme failed to raise testosterone levels or increase muscle strength or mass – in spite of increased levels of androstenedione – compared with a placebo (Brown *et al*, 2000).

What are the side effects?
Studies have found that prohormones increase oestrogen, which can lead to gynecomastia (male breast development) and decrease HDL (high density lipoproteins or 'good' cholesterol) levels (King *et al*, 1999). Reduced HDL carries a greater heart disease risk. Other side effects include acne, enlarged prostate and water retention. Some

supplements include anti-oestrogen substances, such as chrysin (dihydroxyflavone), to counteract the side effects, but there is no evidence that they work either (Brown *et al*, 2000).

Verdict

Prohormones are highly controversial supplements and, despite the rigorous marketing, there is no research to prove the testoster-one-building claims. They are on the World Anti-Doping Agency's prohibited list (WADA, 2014). All sports governing bodies athletic associations, including the International Olympic Committee (IOC), ban prohormones.

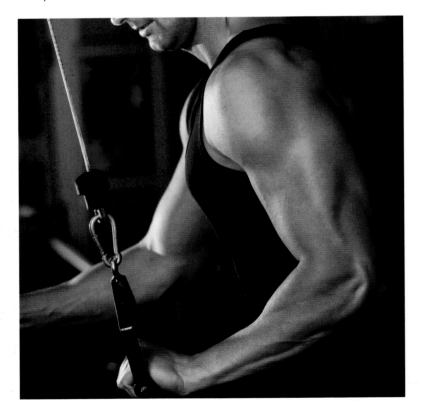

DEFINITION OF A SPORTS DRINK

A sports drink is officially defined by the European Food Safety Agency (EFSA) as a 'carbohydrate-electrolyte solution' containing between 80 to 350 kcal/l and at least 75 per cent of the energy should be derived from carbohydrates which induce a high glycaemic response (such as glucose, glucose polymers and sucrose). In addition these drinks must contain between 20 mmol/l (460 mg/l) and 50 mmol/l (1,150 mg/l) of sodium and have an osmolality between 200 and 330 mOsm/kg water.

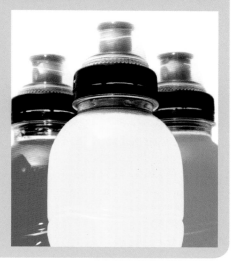

SPORTS DRINKS HEALTH CLAIMS

The European Food Safety Agency (EFSA, 2011) permits only two health claims for sports drinks, which are:
• Enhancement of water absorption during exercise
• Maintenance of endurance performance.

SPORTS DRINKS

There are two categories of 'sports drinks': those that meet the legal definition of a sports drink (isotonic drinks and dual-energy source drinks) and those that fall outside the legal definition but are nevertheless marketed to athletes and regular exercisers (lite sports drinks).

LITE SPORTS DRINKS ('LOW CALORIE', 'HYDRATION', 'ELECTROLYTE' OR 'FITNESS' DRINKS)

What's in them?
This category of drinks is not strictly speaking a sports drink category as it is too low in energy (calories) and carbohydrate to meet the legal definition. These types of drink provide between 0 and 40 g sugar per litre (0–4 per cent sugar), which is about half that of most isotonic sports drinks, along with 400–500 mg sodium per litre. They may also contain other electrolytes (potassium, magnesium, chloride), flavourings, preservatives, colours and sweeteners. Electrolyte tablets contain higher levels of sodium – around 700 mg/l once dissolved in water, but provide no sugar or calories.

All of the drinks in this category are considered 'hypotonic', which means they contain a lower concentration of dissolved particles (sugars and electrolytes) than the body's fluids. They will be absorbed slightly faster than plain water, but slower than isotonic drinks.

How do they work?
In the context of maintaining hydration status, sodium is the most important electrolyte as it helps to stimulate thirst, improve fluid palatability and promote fluid retention. The sugars in these drinks increase the rate at which fluids empty from the stomach, which means they may provide faster rehydration compared with plain water.

What is the evidence?
There have been no studies looking at the effects of hypotonic drinks on performance. However, according to the International Olympic Committee consensus conference, if you're exercising for less than two hours and sweat losses are not excessive, extra electrolytes will not benefit performance (Shirreffs and Sawka, 2011). Contrary to popular belief, electrolytes do not speed fluid delivery (Noakes, 2012; Sawka et al, 2007). Instead, they promote water retention and stimulate thirst. The amount of sugar (and calories) is very low (or, in some cases, zero) so this drinks category will not provide significant amounts of fuel nor increase substantially your endurance.

What are the side effects?

Adverse effects are highly unlikely.

Verdict

The main appeal of these drinks is probably their taste and convenience. As they are sweetened and flavoured, they may make you drink more freely. In other words, they may increase your desire to drink, so you're less likely to get dehydrated during your workout. Electrolyte tablets may be useful when sweat losses are very high and you need rapid sodium replacement, e.g. in hot humid conditions.

MAKE YOUR OWN 'LITE' DRINK

For a calorie-free drink, simply add a dash of sugar-free cordial or squash to your water bottle. For a 2–3 per cent sugar drink, add 50 ml cordial or 65 ml squash to a 1-litre water bottle and top up with water. This provides around 20–30 g sugar per litre. If you're planning to exercise at a high intensity for longer than two hours add 1.25–2.5 g (¼–½ teaspoon) of ordinary salt. This will provide 500–1150 mg of sodium.

WHAT ARE ELECTROLYTES?

Electrolytes are mineral salts that carry an electrical charge ('ions'). They are formed when minerals dissolve and separate in water. The main ones are sodium, chloride, and potassium; others include magnesium, calcium and phosphate. They help to regulate fluid balance between different body compartments (for example, the amount of fluid inside and outside cells) and the volume of fluid in the bloodstream. The water movement is controlled by the concentration of electrolytes on either side of the cell membrane. For example, an increase in the concentration of sodium outside a cell will cause water to move to it from inside the cell. Similarly, a drop in sodium concentration will cause water to move from the outside to the inside of the cell. Potassium draws water across a membrane, so a high potassium concentration inside cells increases the cell's water content.

SPORTS DRINKS (ISOTONIC DRINKS)

What's in them?

Isotonic drinks contain between 40 and 80 g sugars per litre, along with 400–500 mg sodium. They may also contain other electrolytes (e.g. potassium, chloride and magnesium), sweeteners, preservatives, colours and vitamins. The sugars may include glucose, sucrose, fructose and maltodextrin. Isotonic means they contain the same concentration of dissolved particles (sugar and electrolytes) as body fluids, which promotes quicker hydration compared with plain water.

How do they work?

The main benefit of isotonic sports drinks is their sugar content. Sugar speeds the absorption of water, tops up blood sugar levels and provides extra fuel for intense exercise lasting over an hour. The other selling point is their sodium content, which increases the urge to drink, aids water retention and (some say) improves the drink's taste. But, contrary to popular belief, sodium does not speed water absorption and is not necessary for most activities lasting less than two hours. The other electrolytes and vitamins in the drink have no immediate effect on your performance – they just make it a bit 'healthier'!

What is the evidence?

The general consensus of studies suggests that consuming carbohydrate can improve performance during endurance exercise lasting longer than 60–70 minutes (Colombani et al, 2013; Temesi et al, 2011; Vandenbogaerde et al, 2011). By providing the working muscles with additional fuel it is possible to reduce the rate of glycogen depletion and delay fatigue. The optimal amount is 30–60 g per hour for activities between one and three hours, or 60–90 g for activities longer than three hours. You can get 30 g carbohydrate by drinking 500 ml (18 fl oz) of a 6 per cent sports drink over the course of an hour, or 750 ml (26 fl oz) of a 4 per cent sports drink.

Consuming electrolytes (sodium) is unnecessary unless you're exercising for more than two hours or in hot humid conditions when

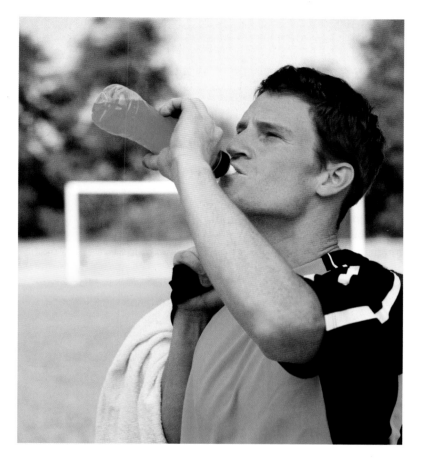

sweat losses are high. Studies suggest that additional sodium will not speed fluid absorption (Gisolfi *et al*, 1995) nor benefit your performance (American College of Sports Medicine, 2007). Sodium increases thirst and makes you want to drink, as well as promoting fluid retention. You have ample sodium in your body so, for most activities under two hours, you should not need to replace sodium sweat losses until after your workout. Electrolyte replacement is only beneficial when sweat losses are high and prolonged, and you lose around 3–4 g sodium (Coyle, 2004).

However, the vast majority of sports drink studies do not reflect competitive real life situations. They often use volunteers in a fasted state, which does not reflect real life situations (most people do not exercise when fasted), and measure 'time to exhaustion' rather than 'time to the finishing line', which would be more meaningful for competitive sports such as swimming, running and cycling. So, it's important to experiment with different formulations, including homemade sports drinks in training to find out what works best for you.

What are the side effects?

If you're exercising to lose weight or prevent weight gain, be mindful of the calorie content. These drinks supply around 280 kcal per litre (or 140 kcal per 500 ml bottle) so unless you are exercising at a high intensity you may end up consuming more calories than you burn.

Verdict

Isotonic sports drinks may benefit your performance if you are exercising at a high intensity for longer than 60 minutes and/or sweating profusely, e.g. in a hot and humid environment. Consuming them during shorter workouts probably won't harm your performance, but you could be consuming something you don't really need. You can obtain similar performance benefits from home-made drinks (e.g. diluted squash or cordial), or real food plus water. In one study at Appalachian State University, bananas were shown to be as effective as a 6 per cent carbohydrate sports drink in fuelling performance in a 75 km cycling time trial (Nieman *et al*, 2011).

MAKE YOUR OWN ISOTONIC DRINK

Add 100 ml cordial or 130 ml squash to a 1-litre water bottle and top up with water. Mix 500 ml apple juice (or your favourite fruit juice) with 500 ml water. If you plan to exercise for more than two hours, or consume the drink after exercise, then add 1.25–2.5 g (¼–½ teaspoon) of ordinary salt. This will provide 500–1150 mg of sodium.

SPORTS DRINKS (DUAL ENERGY SOURCE DRINKS)

What's in them?

This category of sports drinks contains two types of carbohydrate: glucose (or maltodextrin) and fructose in a ratio of 2 to 1. They may also contain sodium, preservatives, flavouring and colouring. The typical sugar content is 7–9 g/100 ml, which makes them isotonic (containing the same concentration of dissolved particles (sugar and electrolytes) as body fluids).

How do they work?

They supply a higher amount of sugars than ordinary isotonic drinks, which will help spare your muscle glycogen stores and increase your endurance. The combination of fructose with glucose or maltodextrin (a short chain of glucose molecules made from corn starch), as opposed to glucose only, allows the body to absorb the sugars more rapidly and therefore deliver them to the muscles at a faster rate than ordinary isotonic drinks. This would be advantageous when you are exercising at high intensities for prolonged periods (2½ hours or longer) and therefore burning glucose at a high rate.

Normally, the body cannot absorb more than about 60 g glucose per hour during endurance exercise. Any excess sits in the stomach longer, requiring dilution before it can pass to the intestine where it is absorbed. This can result in stomach discomfort during exercise. But combining glucose with fructose means that the body can absorb more sugars per minute because each sugar has its own 'transporter' that takes it from the intestines to the bloodstream. Thus you can utilise the two different transporters instead of one and overcome the problem of glucose saturation.

What is the evidence?

Studies have shown that consuming a combination of fructose and glucose (or maltodextrin) during high-intensity prolonged exercise increases the speed of sugar delivery to the muscles compared with glucose alone – up to 1.5 g/minute, or 90 g per hour (Wallis *et al*, 2005). One study suggests that 78 g/hour may be the optimal dose (Smith *et al*, 2013). The drinks may also help reduce perceived fatigue (Rowlands *et al*, 2008).

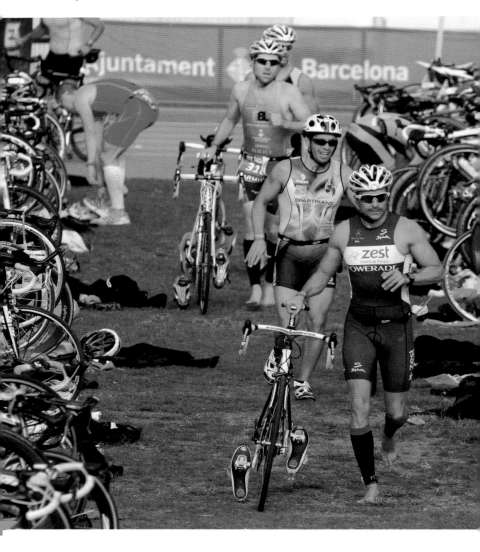

There is promising evidence that these drinks improve your performance. Researchers at Birmingham University found that when cyclists consumed a 2:1 glucose:fructose drink during three hours of cycling, they completed a one-hour time trial 8 per cent faster compared with drinking either water or a glucose-only sports drink (Currell and Jeukendrup, 2008). Other studies have showed improved performance in a 100 km time trial (Triplett *et al*, 2010) and long distance mountain bike events (Rowlands *et al*, 2012).

Are there any side effects?
The drinks may cause mild stomach discomfort in some individuals during training.

Verdict
If you are doing high-intensity endurance activities lasting more than 2½ hours, for example triathlon, cycling or ultra-distance running, where glycogen depletion would be a limiting factor, then dual energy source drinks may help improve your performance and endurance. However, they provide no advantage for lower-intensity exercise (e.g. moderate- or slow-pace running) or anything less than 2½ hours.

MAKE YOUR OWN DUAL ENERGY SOURCE DRINK

Mix 60 g of glucose (or a mixture of glucose and maltodextrin) and 30 g of fructose in 1 litre of water. Add a dash of sugar-free squash to flavour if you like. If this tastes too sweet or you find that it is too concentrated for you (or sits heavily in your stomach), experiment with different amounts and ratios to find what suits you best. Fructose is sweeter than glucose so you may prefer to mix with more maltodextrin than glucose to get the right balance of sweetness.

As you will be exercising longer than 2½ hours, sodium will be beneficial so add 1.25–2.5 g (¼–½ teaspoon) of ordinary salt. This will provide 500–1150 mg of sodium.

SPORTS CONFECTIONERY

What are they?
These products include beans, blocks, jellies and chews. They comprise essentially sugar (sucrose, maltodextrin), but may also contain small amounts of sodium, caffeine and vitamins.

How do they work?
Sports confectionery provides a convenient option for consuming carbohydrate during high-intensity endurance exercise. One serving provides approximately 25 g sugar, enough fuel for about 45-60 minutes of high-intensity activity.

What's the evidence?
A study funded by Jelly Bean undertaken by University College Davis in California found that Sports Beans® jelly beans were equally effective as popular carbohydrate supplements (sports drinks and gels) in maintaining blood sugar levels and improving exercise performance (Campbell *et al*, 2008). Athletes achieved faster times in cycling trials with carbohydrate supplements than they did while consuming only water. As with energy bars and gels, any form of high GI carbohydrate will help improve your endurance during high-intensity exercise lasting longer than one hour.

Are there any side effects?
Some of the products are sticky and may increase the risk of tooth decay so make sure you rinse your mouth well with water after eating them. If you don't drink enough water, they can cause stomach discomfort.

Verdict
If you're exercising at a high intensity for longer than an hour, then sports confectionery may be a convenient way of ingesting extra sugar (and an alternative to gels and bars) to help maintain your blood sugar and spare muscle glycogen. As a general rule, aim for 30-60 g sugar/hour (1-2 servings). Experiment with different doses

and timings (e.g. half a serving every 20 or 30 minutes). Consume with water to avoid gastrointestinal discomfort, but do not wash down with a sports drink otherwise you may consume too much carbohydrate.

Real food alternatives: Try dried fruit such as raisins, dates, pineapple or mango. A study by researchers at the University of California Davis found that people who consumed raisins were able to complete a 5-km time trial faster than those who had only water (Too *et al*, 2012).

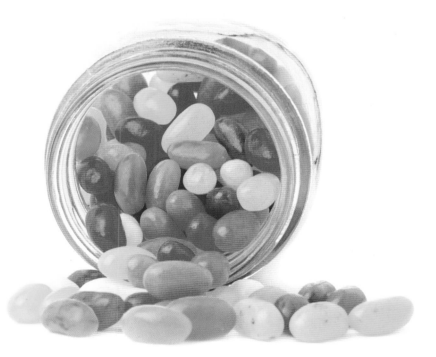

SPORTS RECOVERY DRINKS

What's in them?
Recovery drinks contain a mixture of carbohydrate and protein. The carbohydrate usually comprises sugar and maltodextrin, and the protein may be whey or a mixture of whey, casein and soy.

How do they work?
Consuming protein with carbohydrate stimulates muscle protein synthesis (MPS i.e. muscle repair and growth) and glycogen replenishment, and therefore speeds recovery to a greater extent than carbohydrate or protein alone.

What is the evidence?
The amounts and ratios of carbohydrate to protein vary between brands but research has shown that a 3:1 or 4:1 ratio of carbohydrate to protein promotes the most rapid glycogen re-fuelling (Phillips *et al*, 2007). You'll need between 1 and 1.5 g of carbohydrate per kilogram of body-weight (Rodriguez *et al*, 2009) but you should adjust this depending on the intensity and duration of your workout. After long intense endurance sessions when you've depleted significant amounts of glycogen, you'll need more carbohydrate than after shorter or intermittent workouts. The optimal amount of protein that promotes MPS is 15–25 g (Moore *et al*, 2009). You'll need more (i.e. a dose at the upper end of the range) after strength and power training, and less (i.e. a dose at the lower end of the range) after endurance activities.

Whey is a 'fast-acting' protein which is rapidly digested and absorbed. It also has all the essential amino acids and high levels of

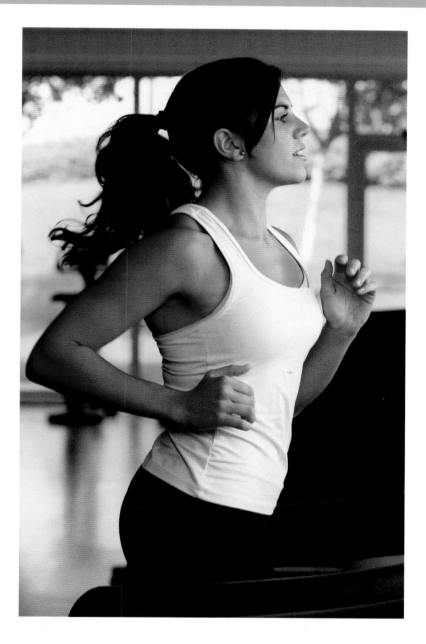

the branched-chain amino acid, leucine, which has been shown to trigger muscle protein synthesis. Studies have shown that whey is superior to casein and soy in promoting muscle repair after resistance exercise (Tang *et al*, 2009; Churchward-Venne *et al*, 2012). However, casein and soy are added to some brands because they are absorbed slower than whey and so provide a 'timed release' of protein to the muscles. The whey delivers quickly while the casein and soy provide a more sustained rise in blood levels of amino acids, extending the window for MPS.

Verdict

Recovery drinks may be useful if you're planning to exercise again within 24 hours. The 2-hour period after exercise represents an ideal opportunity to maximise muscle recovery and glycogen refuelling because recovery takes place one and a half times faster than normal.

However, if you're not intending to exercise within 24 hours or if you've just done a light (non-depleting) training session, then it's less critical to refuel immediately afterwards. Provided you get your daily protein and carbohydrate (and other nutritional requirements) over the next 24 hours, then you'll recover equally well by your next session.

MAKE YOUR OWN RECOVERY DRINK

600 ml of whole, semi-skimmed or skimmed milk provides the all-important 20 g of high-quality protein along with 30 g of carbohydrate, electrolytes (sodium) and other nutrients. Milk also helps rehydrate the body more effectively than sports drinks (Shirreffs *et al*, 2007).

Alternatively, make your own recovery drink with 600 ml milk and 2 tablespoons (30 g) milkshake powder (add more or less according to the length, intensity and type of exercise).

Or blend 500 ml milk, a banana, 100 ml yogurt, and a scoop (25 g) of milkshake powder (after endurance exercise) or whey protein powder (after strength exercise).

TAURINE

What is it?

Taurine is a non-essential amino acid produced naturally in the body. It is also found in meat, fish, eggs and milk. It is the second most abundant amino acid in muscle tissue. It is sold as a single supplement, but more commonly found as an ingredient in some types of protein drinks, creatine based products and sports drinks. It is marketed to athletes for increasing muscle mass and reducing muscle tissue breakdown during intense exercise.

How does it work?

Taurine has multiple roles in the body, including brain and nervous system function, blood pressure regulation, fat digestion, absorption of fat soluble vitamins and control of blood cholesterol levels. The theory behind this supplement is that it may act in a similar way to insulin, transporting amino acids and sugar from the bloodstream into muscle cells. This would cause an increase in cell volume, triggering protein synthesis and less protein breakdown.

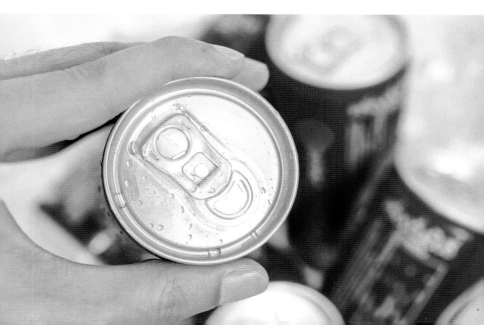

What is the evidence?

Intense exercise depletes taurine levels in the body, but there is no sound research to support the claims for taurine supplements. In a randomised double blind crossover trial, US researchers found no difference in either strength or muscular endurance in athletes following consumption of 500 ml sugar-free Red Bull energy drink (containing taurine and caffeine) compared with a drink containing caffeine (without taurine) or a placebo (without caffeine or taurine) (Eckerson *et al*, 2013).

Similarly, another study by a different team of researchers measured no difference in endurance cycling performance following consumption of an energy drink containing taurine (and caffeine) compared with cola (containing caffeine) or a placebo (Phillips *et al*, 2013).

A Canadian study found that when trained cyclists consumed taurine prior to a time trial, there was no difference in their performance compared with a placebo (Rutherford *et al*, 2010).

Are there any side effects?

It is harmless in the amounts found in protein and creatine supplements. Very high doses (more than 3 g) of single supplements may cause toxicity.

Verdict

As you can obtain it from food (animal protein sources) there appears to be no convincing reason to recommend taking taurine supplements for athletic performance or muscle gain.

TESTOSTERONE BOOSTERS

What are they?
These include tribulus terrestris (a flowering plant), horny goat weed (a leafy plant) and zinc. They are marketed as natural alternatives to anabolic steroids.

How do they work?
Manufacturers claim that the phytochemicals in the plants increase testosterone production and therefore increase muscle mass and strength as well as boosting libido.

What is the evidence?
There is no evidence supporting the claims for tribulus terrestris or horny goat weed. A four-week study of 21 healthy young men failed to find any measurable differences in testosterone levels between those taking a tribulus terrestris supplement and a placebo group

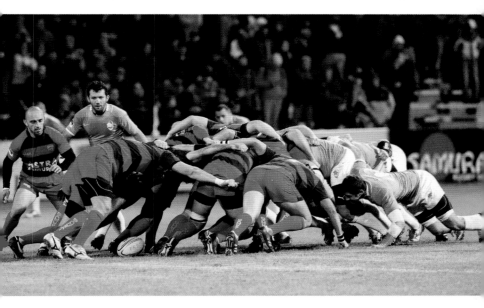

(Neychev and Mitev, 2005). Similarly, a study of 22 Australian elite rugby players found no difference in testosterone levels, nor any improvement in strength or body composition after five weeks of supplementation with tribulus terrestris compared with a placebo (Rogerson *et al*, 2007).

Despite the manufacturers' claims, there have been no studies on horny goat weed and testosterone levels in humans – only studies with rats!

Zinc supplements do not raise testosterone levels unless you have a deficiency, i.e. abnormally low testosterone levels (see 'ZMA', page 126). By correcting the deficiency, you may notice a short-term improvement in strength and muscle mass.

Are there any side effects?
Tribulus supplements are unlikely to produce side effects. However, they are contra-indicated for people with breast or prostate cancer.

Verdict
Despite the claims, testosterone boosters do not increase testosterone, improve muscle mass or enhance athletic performance. Although some manufacturers claim tribulus terrestris will not lead to a positive drug test, others have suggested it may increase the urinary testosterone/epitestosterone (T/E) ratio, which may place athletes at risk of a positive drug test. So you should avoid anything containing this supplement if you compete in a drug-tested sport.

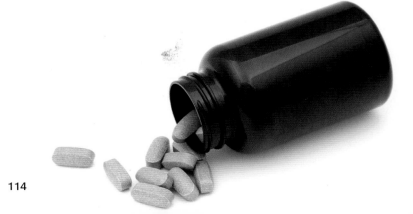

VITAMIN C

What is it?

Vitamin C is a water-soluble vitamin found naturally in fresh fruit and vegetables.

How does it work?

Vitamin C is required for the formation of connective tissue and certain hormones (e.g. adrenaline), which are produced during exercise. It is involved in the formation of red blood cells, which enhances iron

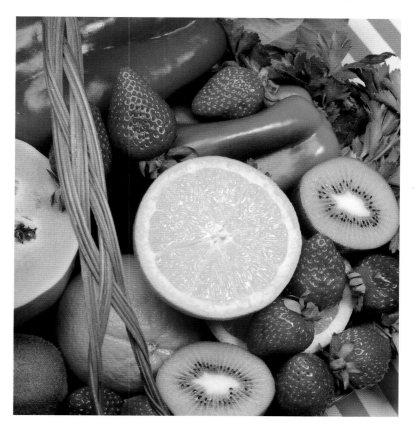

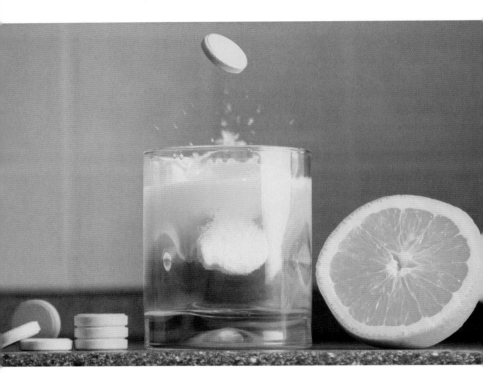

absorption, and is a powerful antioxidant, which can protect against cell damage. Thus, supplementation may help enhance recovery from exercise and help protect against illnesses and injuries.

What is the evidence?

There's little evidence that vitamin C supplementation improves performance in athletes who are not deficient in the vitamin. In fact, rather than improve exercise performance, high doses (more than 1000 mg) of vitamin C may impair it.

In a double blind randomised study, athletes who took vitamin C supplements (1000 g/day) experienced a reduction in endurance capacity after eight weeks (Gomez-Cabrera *et al*, 2008). That's because supplements prevented muscle cell adaptations (e.g. an increase in enzyme production) to exercise, resulting in no improvement in aerobic capacity.

Norwegian researchers found that people who took high dose supplements of vitamin C (1000 mg) and vitamin E (235 mg) for 11 weeks gained no performance benefit compared with those taking a placebo (Paulsen *et al*, 2013). Those taking the supplements produced fewer extra mitochondria, which are needed to improve endurance. The researchers concluded that vitamins C and E should be used with caution as they may 'blunt' the way muscles respond to exercise.

A review of studies concluded that vitamin C supplementation reduced the benefits of training and resulted in slower recovery and strength gains (Adams *et al*, 2014).

On the other hand, lower doses of vitamin C may help protect against infection during periods of heavy training or after high-intensity endurance events. One study found a reduced incidence in upper respiratory tract infections in ultra-marathon runners after taking 600 mg vitamin C for 21 days prior to the race. In another, ultra-marathon runners who took daily vitamin C supplements seven days prior to a race had lower levels of stress hormones following the race, which suggests greater protection against infection (Peters *et al*, 2001).

Are there any side effects?
Doses higher than 3 g per day may cause gastro-intestinal discomfort and diarrhoea.

Verdict
There is little justification for vitamin C supplementation. High doses (more than 1000 mg) may blunt the muscles' ability to adapt to exercise and hinder rather than help your performance. Lower doses (less than 1000 mg) may be beneficial during periods of stress or intensified training, but are unlikely to benefit your performance at other times. Aim to get your daily vitamin C from your diet rather than supplements. Best food sources include berries, dark green leafy vegetables, citrus fruit and peppers.

VITAMIN D

What is it?

Vitamin D is a fat-soluble vitamin. The main source comes from exposure to ultraviolet B (UVB) radiation, but it can also be obtained from oily fish, egg yolk and fortified foods (e.g. cereals and margarine).

How does it work?

Vitamin D promotes calcium absorption. It is needed for optimal bone mass, but also for muscular performance and immune function. Low levels may reduce muscle function and strength and may also increase the risk of injury and illness – all of which would have a detrimental effect on your training and performance (Hamilton,

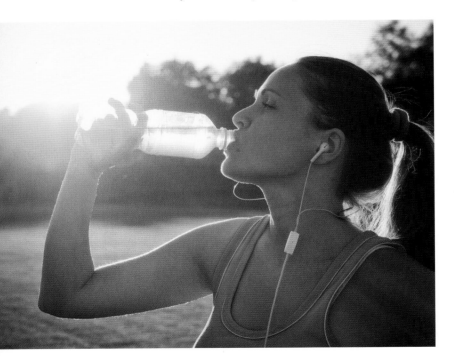

2011; Larson-Meyer and Willis, 2010; Halliday *et al*, 2011). Getting adequate levels of vitamin D whether from sun exposure or diet is, therefore, important for optimal performance.

What is the evidence?

Several studies have observed a correlation between vitamin D status and athletic performance (Larson-Meyer and Willis, 2010). It appears low levels are associated with reduced performance while high levels may enhance performance. A review of studies has highlighted a seasonal variation in performance (Cannell *et al*, 2009). It revealed that performance peaks in the summer months (when vitamin D levels peak), declines in winter months (when vitamin D levels decline), and reaches its lowest point when vitamin D levels are at their lowest. Peak athletic performance seems to occur when vitamin D levels approach those obtained by natural, full-body, summer sun exposure, which is around 50 ng/ml.

Several studies suggest that vitamin D deficiency is widespread among athletes, particularly those in northern latitudes who train mainly indoors or get little sun exposure, or who do not consume

HOW TO GET ENOUGH VITAMIN D

There are only three categories of foods that contain significant amounts of vitamin D: eggs, liver and oily fish. Vitamin D is found only in the yolk of the egg so do use the whole egg when making omelettes, or scrambled eggs. Each of the following provides 5 ug:

- 3 eggs
- ½ tsp (2.5 ml) cod liver oil
- 100 g tinned sardines
- 60 g mackerel
- 70 g salmon
- 170 g tinned tuna (in oil).

vitamin D-rich foods (Larson-Meyer and Willis, 2010; Lovell, 2008; Meier *et al*, 2004). One study of NCAA athletes at the University of California suggested 33 per cent were deficient (Villacis *et al*, 2014).

According to another study, as many as 62 per cent of UK athletes have insufficient or deficient levels of serum vitamin D, defined as less than 50 ng/ml (Close *et al*, 2013). After taking vitamin D supplements for eight weeks there was a significant improvement in vertical jump height and 10 m sprint times compared with those given a placebo. In other words, correcting vitamin D deficiency through supplementation appears to improve athletic performance.

Are there any side effects?
The safe upper limit is 25 micrograms (µg) or 1000 International Units (IU) in the UK, and 50 µg (2000 IU) in the US. Toxicity is rare but may include weakness, muscle pain, high blood pressure, nausea, irregular heartbeat and thirst. This may occur in doses over 250 µg (10,000 IU).

Verdict
It is clear that low levels of vitamin D may impair performance. However, supplements would only benefit athletic performance if you are deficient (Powers *et al*, 2011). You should endeavour to maintain healthy blood levels of vitamin D (ideally more than 75 nmol/l) whether from sun exposure or diet. Aim for 15 minutes' sun exposure a day with face and arms uncovered from April to September, otherwise supplements may be a good idea during the winter months when levels of vitamin D are low (IOC, 2011; Halliday *et al*, 2011).

If you think you may be at risk of vitamin D deficiency, you should consult your doctor who may recommend a simple blood test to determine whether you would benefit from vitamin D supplements. If you decide to take supplements, opt for Vitamin D3 rather than D2 – this form is used more effectively by the body.

There's debate about the ideal level of vitamin D needed to prevent deficiency. There's no RDA in the UK, but the US recommend intakes of 15 µg/day (600 IU) and the EU recommend 5 µg daily.

VITAMIN E

What is it?

Vitamin E is a fat-soluble vitamin found in nuts, seeds, plant oils, oily fish, avocados and egg yolks. It comprises a group of eight different compounds, which collectively help protect the body from oxidative damage.

How does it work?

Intense exercise creates an imbalance between damaging reactive oxygen species (free radicals – see page 24) and the body's antioxidants which protect against them, leading to the condition of oxidative stress. Vitamin E functions primarily as an antioxidant, preventing the oxidation of fatty acids in cell membranes and protecting cells from damage. It is thought that vitamin E supplements help reduce oxidative stress during exercise and promote faster recovery.

What is the evidence?

Early studies indicated that vitamin E supplementation reduced oxidative stress, although it had no immediate effect on performance (Rokitzki et al, 1994).

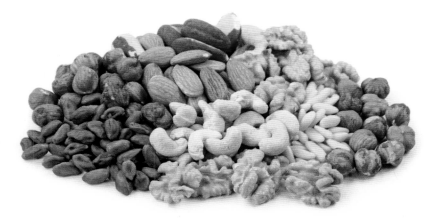

However, more recent studies have shown that supplementation may reduce training adaptations and result in decreased performance (see also 'antioxidants', page 24). For example, triathletes who took vitamin E supplements (800 IU) daily for two months performed no better than those who took a placebo (Nieman *et al*, 2004). Although blood levels of vitamin E were higher, this did not reduce markers of oxidative stress nor translate into any improvement in performance. Similarly, another study found that eight weeks of vitamin E supplementation did not reduce markers of oxidative stress nor improve exercise performance (Gaeini *et al*, 2006). And more recently, Norwegian researchers showed that supplementation with vitamins E and C did not improve endurance performance compared with a placebo (Paulsen *et al*, 2013). This is because the vitamin supplements interfered with exercise-induced cell-signalling in cell muscle fibres.

Are there any side effects?
Vitamin E, despite being a fat-soluble vitamin and capable of being stored, appears safe at levels 50 times higher than the RDA.

Verdict
Taking high doses of vitamin E supplements will not confer any performance advantage and may even reduce the fitness gains from your workouts. Like vitamin C, high doses of vitamin E appear to blunt the training response. Aim to get your vitamin E from a healthy diet instead of supplements. Rich sources include nuts, seeds, avocados and egg yolks.

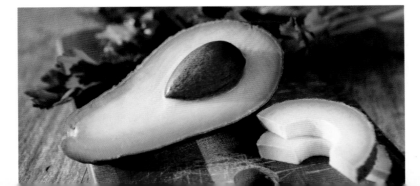

WHEY PROTEIN

What is it?

Whey protein is derived from milk (as the by-product of cheese production) and provides a balanced source of all nine essential amino acids, including the branched-chain amino acids, leucine, isoleucine and valine. There are three types of whey supplements:

- Whey protein concentrate – produced by ultrafiltration of whey, generally contains about 80 per cent protein (the remainder being lactose, fat and water).
- Whey protein isolate – produced by a variety of membrane filtration or ion-exchange techniques that remove almost all the lactose and fat, and generally contains more than 90 per cent protein.
- Whey protein hydrolysates – produced by enzymatic hydrolysis of whey concentrate or whey isolate, which 'pre-digests' the protein by separating peptide bonds; so it is digested and absorbed faster.

How does it work?

Whey is digested quickly and rapidly absorbed in the intestine. It may also help enhance the immune function thanks to its high content of glutamine. It provides high levels of leucine, which is both a key signal molecule for initiation of muscle protein synthesis (MPS) and an important substrate for muscle protein.

What is the evidence?

In studies where athletes were already consuming adequate amounts of protein in their diet, taking additional protein in the form of supplements before and after their workouts made no difference to muscle synthesis or strength (Weisgarber et al, 2012).

Whey supplements may help increase muscle synthesis following resistance training. In one study those consuming 20 g of whey supplement before and after resistance exercise had greater increases in muscle mass and muscle strength over ten weeks compared with those consuming a placebo (Willoughby *et al*, 2007). Another study found that when athletes consumed a whey supplement immediately before and after a training session they could perform more reps and lift heavier weights 24 hours and 48 hours after the workout compared with those taking a placebo (Hoffman *et al*, 2008).

However, consuming any high-quality protein source immediately after resistance training will also promote muscle repair and growth (Tipton *et al*, 2004). Compared with casein or soy, whey supplements may be a better option in the immediate post-exercise period as whey is absorbed quicker, but there is no evidence that it results in greater muscle growth over 24 hours (Tang *et al*, 2009).

Whey may also help boost immunity. Researchers found that those who consumed whey supplements following a 40-km cycling time trial experienced a smaller drop in glutathione levels, which is linked with lowered immunity (Middleton, Jelen and Bell, 2004).

Are there any side effects?

An excessive intake of protein, whether from food or supplements, is not harmful but offers no health or performance advantage. Concerns about excess protein harming the liver and kidneys or causing calcium loss from the bones have been disproved.

Verdict

If you are getting enough protein from food, there's probably little point in taking supplements. You may prefer to drink milk (which contains whey naturally) as studies have shown that it is just as effective in promoting muscle synthesis after resistance training as supplements. Athletes who consumed milk gained more muscle than those consuming soy protein drinks during a 12-week resistance training programme (Hartman *et al*, 2007).

But if you have higher-than-average requirements, whey protein may be a convenient way of adding protein to your diet. It may also be useful for vegetarians who may not get enough protein from animal sources. Whey protein drinks and bars may also be a convenient way of getting your protein when you're out and about. However, whey supplements are generally more expensive than real food (such as milk).

As whey is quickly digested, supplements may be helpful for promoting recovery after exercise if you plan to train again within 24 hours. However, it won't necessarily produce faster or greater muscle gains than real food sources of whey, such as milk, yoghurt and cheese. Most studies have compared whey with carbohydrate, casein or soy supplements, and not with real food.

HOW MUCH PROTEIN DO ATHLETES NEED?

It is widely accepted that athletes have higher protein requirements than the general population. This extra protein is needed to repair damaged muscle cells after intense exercise, as well as to build new muscle proteins (Rodriguez *et al*, 2009; Phillips, 2007; Campbell *et al*, 2007). The exact amount of protein necessary for muscle building has been hotly debated for many years but scientists currently recommend an intake between 1.3 and 1.8 g protein/kg body weight per day for athletes generally; with intakes at the higher end of this range (1.6-1.8 g) for strength and power athletes (Phillips and van Loon, 2011). This translates to 112-126 g daily for a 70 kg person, considerably more than the Guideline Daily Amount (GDA) for the general population, which is 45 g for women and 55 g for men.

WHAT IS THE IDEAL POST-WORKOUT PROTEIN INTAKE?

Canadian researchers found that 20-25 g is the optimal level for muscle growth immediately after a weights workout (Moore *et al*, 2009). When athletes consumed less than 20 g they gained less muscle; when they consumed more than this amount they experienced no further muscle gains. However, it's best to think of 20-25 g as a ballpark figure. If you weigh more than 85 kg (the weight of the athletes in the study) then you will need more, if you weigh less than 85 kg you may need less. You can get 20 g protein from 85 g (3 oz) steak or chicken, 3 eggs or 500 ml (18 fl oz) milk.

ZMA

What is it?

ZMA (the acronym for zinc and magnesium aspartate) is a supplement that combines zinc, magnesium, vitamin B6 and aspartate in a specific formula. It is claimed that ZMA can boost testosterone production, increase strength and improve muscle mass, and promote recovery after exercise.

How does it work?

Both zinc and magnesium play critical roles in performance. Zinc is needed for growth, cell reproduction and testosterone production. In theory, a deficiency may reduce the body's anabolic hormone levels and adversely affect muscle mass and strength. Magnesium assists with muscle contractions and energy metabolism. Apart from being used in the production of energy, magnesium might also help performance by reducing accumulation of lactic acid and reducing the perception of fatigue during strenuous exercise through its action on the nervous system. A magnesium deficiency may reduce endurance.

What is the evidence?

Both zinc and magnesium deficiencies can impair performance (Nielsen and Lukaski, 2006). It is feasible that ZMA supplementation corrects underlying zinc and/or magnesium deficiencies, thus 'normalising' various body processes and improving testosterone levels. This is supported by one study, which found ZMA increased testosterone and strength in a group of football players (Brilla and Conte, 2000). However, this was a small study with a high dropout rate and has not been replicated since.

A more rigorous randomised, double-blind study with 42 experienced weight-trainers found that supplementation with ZMA for eight weeks failed to increase testosterone levels, strength, muscle mass, anaerobic capacity or muscular endurance compared with a placebo (Wilborn et al, 2004).

Are there any side effects?

High levels of zinc – more than 50 mg – can interfere with the absorption of iron and other minerals, leading to iron deficiency. High doses of magnesium can cause diarrhoea and interfere with calcium absorption.

Verdict

By bringing deficient mineral status up to 'normal' levels, you may see an increase in health or performance. However, if you are not deficient, taking additional quantities of zinc and magnesium probably won't help you gain muscle mass or get stronger. It cannot be recommended for 'boosting testosterone' or improving performance. You can obtain zinc from whole grains, including wholemeal bread, nuts, beans and lentils. Magnesium is found in nuts, whole grains, green leafy vegetables, fruit and milk.

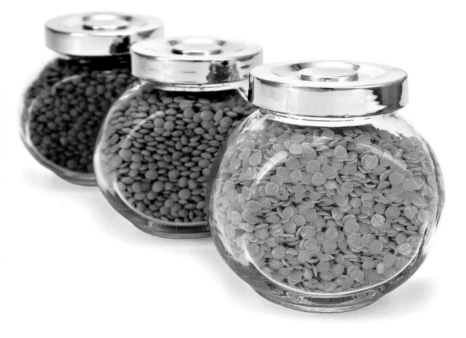

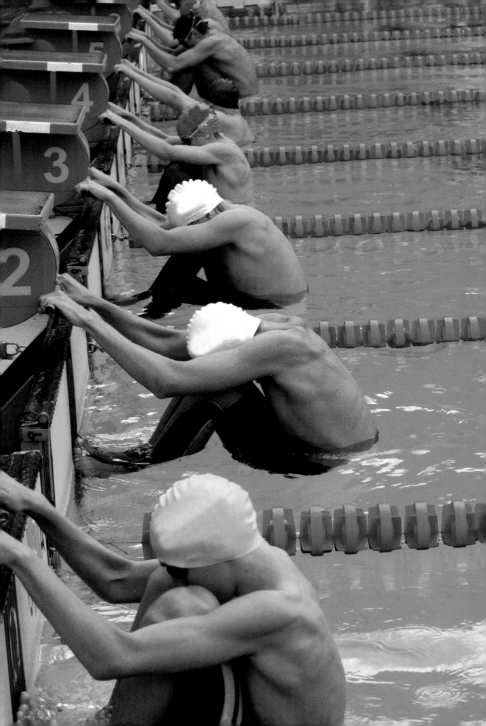

REFERENCES

Adams, R.B., Egbo, K.N., Demmig-Adams, B. (2014). 'High-dose vitamin C supplements diminish the benefits of exercise in athletic training and disease prevention', *Nutrition & Food Science*, 44 (2), pp. 95–101.

American College of Sports Medicine, Sawka, M.N., *et al.* (2007). 'American College of Sports Medicine Position stand. Exercise and fluid replacement', *Med. Sci. Sports. Exerc*, 39 pp. 377–390.

American College of Sports Medicine, Rodriguez, N.R., Di Marco, N. M. and Langley, S. (2009) 'American College of Sports Medicine position stand: Nutrition and athletic performance', *Med. Sci. Sports Exerc.*, pp. 709-731.

Anderson, M., *et al.* (2000). 'Improved 2000 m rowing performance in competitive oarswomen after caffeine ingestion', *Int. J. Sport Nutr.* 10, 464–475.

Anderson, M.J., *et al.* (2001). 'Effect of glycerol-induced hyperhydration on thermoregulation and metabolism during exercise in heat.', *Int. J. Sport Nutr. Exerc. Metab.* 1(3), 315–333.

Antonio, J., and Ciccone, V. (2013). 'The effects of pre versus post workout supplementation of creatine monohydrate on body composition and strength', *Int. J. Soc. Sports. Nutr.,* 10, 36.

Areces, F., *et al.* (2014). 'A 7-day oral supplementation with branched-chain amino acids was ineffective to prevent muscle damage during a marathon', *Amino Acids*, 46 (5), 1169–1176.

Armstrong, L.E., *et al.* (2005). 'Fluid, electrolyte and renal indices of hydration during 11 days of controlled caffeine consumption', *Int. J. Sport Nutr. Exerc. Metab.*, 15, 252-265.

Bailey, S.J., et al. (2009). 'Dietary nitrate supplementation reduces the O2 cost of low-intensity exercise and enhances tolerance to high-intensity exercise in humans.', J. Appl. Physiol., 107(4), 1144–1155.

Ballantyne, C.S., et al. (2000). 'The acute effects of androstenedione supplementation in healthy young males.' J. Appl. Physiol., 25(1), 68–78.

Ballard, S.L., Wellborn-Kim, J.J., Clauson, K.A. (2010). 'Effects of Commercial Energy Drink Consumption on Athletic Performance and Body Composition', Physician and Sports Medicine, 38(1), 107–117.

Barnett, C., et al. (1994). 'Effect of L-carnitine supplementation on muscle and blood carnitine content and lactate accumulation during high-intensity sprint cycling.', Int. J. Sport Nutr., 4(3), 280–288.

Barrett, B., et al. (2010) 'Echinacea for treating the common cold: a randomized trial' Annals of Internal Medicine 2010, 153, 769–777.

Beis, L.Y., et al. (2011). 'The effects of creatine and glycerol hyperhydration on running economy in well trained endurance runners.' J. Int. Soc. Sports Nutr., 16;8(1), 24

Bell, D.G., et al. (2001). 'Effect of caffeine and ephedrine ingestion on anaerobic exercise performance', Med. Sci. Sport Exerc., 33(8), 1399–1403.

Bescos, R., et al. (2012). 'The effect of nitric oxide related supplements on human performance', Sports Med., 42(2), 99–117.

Bjelakovic, G., et al. (2012). 'Antioxidant supplements for prevention of mortality in healthy participants and patients with various diseases', Cochrane Database of Systematic Reviews 2012, 3.

Brilla, L.R., and Conte, V., (2000). 'Effects of a novel zinc-magnesium formulation on hormones and strength', J. Exerc. Physiol., [online]. 3(4), 1–15.

Brinkworth, G.D., and Buckley, J.D., (2003). 'Concentrated bovine colostrum protein supplementation reduces the incidence of self-reported symptoms of upper respiratory tract infection in adult males', Eur. J. Nutr., 42, 228–32.

Brinkworth, G.D., *et al.* (2004). 'Effect of bovine colostrum supplementation on the composition of resistance trained and untrained limbs in healthy young men', *Eur. J. Appl. Physiol.,* 91, 53–60.

Broeder, C.E., *et al.* (2000). 'The Andro Project', *Arch. Intern. Med.,* 160(20), 3093–3104.

Brown, G.A., *et al.* (1999). 'Effect of oral DHEA on serum testosterone and adaptations to resistance training in young men.', *J. Appl. Physiol.,* 87, 2274–2283.

Brown, G.A., *et al.* (1999). 'Effect of oral DHEA on serum testosterone and adaptations to resistance training in young men', *J. A. P. Online,* 87(6), 2007–2015.

Brown, G.A., *et al.* (2000). 'Effects of anabolic precursors on serum testosterone concentrations and adaptations to resistance training in young men', *Int. J. Sport Nutr.,* 10, 340–359.

Brownlie, T., *et al.* (2004) 'Tissue iron deficiency without anemia impairs adaptation in endurance capacity after aerobic training in previously untrained women'. *Am. J. Clin. Nutr.,* 79(3):437-43.

Buford, T.W., *et al.* (2007). 'International Society of Sports Nutrition position stand: creatine supplementation and exercise.', *J. Int. Soc. Sports Nutr.,* 4, 6.

Burke, L.M. (2008). 'Caffeine and sports performance.', *Appl. Physiol. Nutr. Metab.,* 33(6), 1319–1334.

Cameron SL, *et al.* (2010) 'Increased blood pH but not performance with sodium bicarbonate supplementation in elite rugby union players'. *Int. J. Sport Nutr. Exerc. Metab.,* 20(4):307-21.

Campbell, C., *et al* (2008) 'Carbohydrate-supplement form and exercise performance.' *Int. J. Sports Nutr. Exerc. Metab.,* 18(2):179-90.

Candow, D.G., *et al.* (2001). 'Effect of glutamine supplementation combined with resistance training in young adults', *Eur. J. Appl. Physiol.,* 86(2), 142–149.

Cannell, J., *et al.* (2009). 'Athletic performance and vitamin D', *Med. Sci. Sports Exerc.,* 41, 1102–1110.

Carr, A. J *et al* (2011), 'Effects of acute alkalosis and acidosis on performance: a meta-analysis,' *Sports Med.* vol. 41(10), pp. 801–14.

Cermak, N.M., *et al.* (2012). 'Nitrate supplementation's improvement of 10 km time trial performance in trained cyclists', *Int. J. Sport Nutr. Exerc. Metab.,* 1, 64–71.

Churchward-Venne, T.A., Burd, N.A., Phillips, S.M. (2012). 'Nutritional regulation of muscle protein synthesis with resistance exercise: strategies to enhance anabolism.', *Nutrition & Metabolism*, 9(1), 40.

Clegg, D.O., *et al.* (2006). 'Glucosamine, chondroitin sulfate, and the two in combination for painful knee osteoarthritis.', *N. Engl. J. Med.,* 23;354(8), 795–808.

Close, G.L., *et al.* (2013). 'Assessment of vitamin D concentration in non-supplemented professional athletes and healthy adults during the winter months in the UK: implications for skeletal muscle function.', *J. Sports. Sci.* 31(4), 344–53.

Coffey, C.S., *et al.* (2004). 'A randomised double-blind placebo-controlled clinical trial of a product containing ephedrine, caffeine, and other ingredients from herbal sources for treatment of overweight and obesity in the absence of lifestyle treatment.' *Int. J. Obes. Relat. Metab. Disord.,* 28(11), 1411–1419.

Colombani, P.C., Mannhart, C., Mettler, S. (2013). 'Carbohydrates and exercise performance in non-fasted athletes: A systematic review of studies mimicking real-life', *Nutrition Journal 2013*, 12, 16.

Cooke, M.B., *et al.* (2014). 'Creatine supplementation post-exercise does not enhance training-induced adaptations in middle to older aged males.' *Eur. J. Appl. Physiol.* 2014 Mar 2016 (Epub ahead of print).

Cooper, R., *et al.* (2012). 'Creatine supplementation with specific view to exercise/sports performance: an update', *J. Int. Soc. Sports Nutr.,* 9, 33.

Crowe, M.J., Weatherson, J.N., Bowden, B.F. (2006). 'Effects of dietary leucine supplementation on exercise performance', *Eur. J. Appl. Physiol.,* 97(6), 664.

Cox, A.J., *et al.* (2008). 'Oral administration of the probiotic Lactobacillus fermentum VRI-003 and mucosal immunity in endurance athletes.', *Br. J. Sports Med.* (Epub: Feb 2013).

Coyle, E.F. (2004). 'Fluid and fuel intake during exercise.' *J. Sports Sci.,* 22(1), 39–55.

Crooks, C.V., *et al.* (2006) 'The effect of bovine colostrum supplementation on salivary IgA in distance runners', *Int. J. Sports Nutr. Exerc. Metab.,* 16(1) pp. 47–64.

Currell, K., and Jeukendrup, A.E. (2008). 'Superior endurance performance with ingestion of multiple transportable carbohydrates.', *Med. Sci .Sports Exerc.,* 40, 275–281.

Davison, G. (2012). 'Bovine colostrum and immune function after exercise.', *Med. Sport Sci. 2012,* 59, 62–9.

Dellavalle, D.M., Haas, J.D. (2013). 'Iron Supplementation Improves Energetic Efficiency in Iron-Depleted Female Rowers.' Med. Sci. Sports Exerc. Nov 2015 (Epub ahead of print).

Derave, W., Ozdemir, M.S., Harris, R.C., *et al.* (2007). 'Beta-alanine supplementation augments muscle carnosine content and attenuates fatigue during repeated isokinetic contraction bouts in trained sprinters.', *J. Appl. Physiol.,* 103, 1736–1743.

Doherty, M., and Smith, P.M. (2004). 'Effects of caffeine ingestion on exercise testing: a meta-analysis', *Int. J. Sport Nutr. Exerc. Metab.,* 14, 626–646.

Donovan, T., *et al.* (2012). 'Beta-alanine improves punch force and frequency in amateur boxers during a simulated contest.', *Int. J. Sport Nutr. Exerc. Metab.,* 22(5), 331–337.

Draeger, C.L., *et al.* (2014). 'Controversies of antioxidant vitamins supplementation in exercise: ergogenic or ergolytic effects in humans?', *J. Int. Soc. Sports Nutr.,* 11, 4.

Driller, M.W., *et al.* (2012) 'The effects of serial and acute NaHCO3 loading in well-trained cyclists'. *J. Strength Cond. Res.,* 26(10), pp.2791–7.

Ducker, K.J., Dawson, B., Wallman, K.E. (2013). 'Effect of beta-alanine supplementation on 800-m running performance.', *Int. J. Sport Nutr. Exerc., Metab.* 23(6), 554–561.

Dulloo, A.G., *et al.* (1999). 'Efficacy of a green tea extract rich in catechin polyphenols and caffeine in increasing 24-h energy expenditure and fat oxidation in humans.', *Am. J. Clin. Nutr.,* 70(6), 1040–1045.

Eckerson, J.M., *et al.* (2013). 'Acute ingestion of sugar-free Red Bull energy drink has no effect on upper body strength and muscular endurance in resistance trained men.', *J. Strength Cond. Res.,* 27(8), 2248–2254.

EFSA. (2011). 'Scientific opinion on the substantiation of health claims related to carbohydrate-electrolyte solutions and reduction in rated perceived exertion/effort during exercise, enhancement of water absorption during exercise and maintenance of endurance performance pursuant to Article 13(1) of Regulation (EC) No 1924/2006', *EFSA Journal,* 9(6), 2211.

Fiala, K.A. *et al.* (2004). 'Rehydration with a caffeinated beverage during the non-exercise periods of 3 consecutive days of a 2-a-day practices', *Int. J. Sport Nutr. Exerc. Metab.,* 14, 419–429.

Forbes, S.C., *et al.* (2007). 'Effect of Red Bull energy drink on repeated Wingate cycle performance and bench-press muscle endurance', *Int. J. Sport Nutr. Exerc. Metab.,* 17(5), 433–444.

Fortmann, S.P., *et al.* (2013). 'Vitamin and Mineral Supplements in the Primary Prevention of Cardiovascular Disease and Cancer: An Updated Systematic Evidence Review for the U.S. Preventive Services Task Force.', *Annals of Internal Medicine.,* 159(12), 824–834.

Gaeini, A.A., Rahnama, N., Hamedinia, M.R. (2006). 'Effects of vitamin E supplementation on oxidative stress at rest and after exercise to exhaustion in athletic students.', *J. Sports Med. Phys. Fitness.,* 46(3), 458–461.

Gant, N., Ali, A., Foskett, A. (2010). 'The Influence of Caffeine and Carbohydrate Coingestion on Simulated Soccer Performance.', *Int. J. Sport Nutr. Exerc. Metab.,* 20, 191–197.

Gaullier, J.M., *et al.* (2005). 'Conjugated linoleic acid supplementation for 1 y reduces body fat mass in healthy overweight humans', *J. Nutr.,* 135, 778–784.

Gebauer, S.K., *et al.* (2006). 'n-3 fatty acid dietary recommendations and food sources to achieve essentiality and cardiovascular benefits.', *Am. J. Clin. Nutr.,* 83, 1526-1535.

Geyer, H., *et al.* (2004). 'Analysis of non-hormonal nutritional supplements for anabolic – androgenic steroids – results of an international study', *Int. J. Sports Med.*, 25(2), 124–129.

Gilchrist, M., Winyard, P.G., Benjamin, N. (2010). 'Dietary nitrate – good or bad?' *Nitric Oxide,* 22, 104-109.

Gisolfi, C.V., *et al.* (1995). 'Effect of sodium concentration in a carbohydrate-electrolyte solution on intestinal absorption', *Med. Sci. Sports Ex.,* 27(10), 1414–1420.

Gleeson, M. (2008). 'Dosing and efficacy of glutamine supplementation in human exercise and sport training.', *J. Nutr.,* 138(10), 2045–2049.

Goldstein, E.R., *et al.* (2010). 'International society of sports nutrition position stand: caffeine and performance', *J. Int. Soc. Sports Nut.,* 7(1), 5.

Gomez-Cabrera, M.C., *et al.* (2008). 'Oral administration of vitamin C decreases muscle mitochondrial biogenesis and hampers training-induced adaptations in endurance performance.', *Am. J. Clin. Nutr.,* 87(1), 142–149.

Goulet, E.D., *et al.* (2006). 'Effect of glycerol-induced hyperhydration on thermoregulatory and cardiovascular functions and endurance performance during prolonged cycling in a 25 degrees C environment.', *Appl. Physiol. Nutr. Metab.,* 31(2), 101–109.

Graham, T.E., Hibbert, E., Sathasivam, P. (1998). 'Metabolic and exercise endurance effects of coffee and caffeine ingestion.', *J. Appl. Physiol.,* 85, 883–889.

Greer, B.K., *et al.* (2007). 'Branched-chain amino acid supplementation and indicators of muscle damage after endurance exercise', *Int. J. Sports Nutr. Exerc. Metab.,* 17, 595–607.

Gregersen, N.T., *et al.* (2009). 'Effect of moderate intakes of different tea catechins and caffeine on acute measures of energy metabolism under sedentary conditions.', *Br. J. Nutr.,* 102(8), 1187–1194.

Grodstein, F., *et al.* (2013). 'Long-Term Multivitamin Supplementation and Cognitive Function in Men: A Randomised Trial.', *Annals of Internal Medicine*, 159(12), 806–814.

Gualano, B., *et al.* (2012). 'In sickness and in health: The widespread application of creatine supplementation.', *Amino Acids*, 43, 519–529.

Halliday, T., *et al.* (2011). 'Vitamin D status relative to diet, lifestyle, injury and illness in college athletes', *Med. Sci. Sports Exerc.*, 43, 335–343.

Hamilton, B. (2011) 'Vitamin D and athletic performance: the potential role of muscle'. Asian J. Sports Med., vol. 2(4), pp. 211–219.

Hao, Q., *et al.* (2011). 'Probiotics for preventing acute upper respiratory tract infections.', *Cochrane Database Syst Rev.*, 7(9).

Harris, R.C., *et al.* (2006). 'The absorption of orally supplied beta-alanine and its effect on muscle carnosine synthesis in human vastus lateralis.', *Amino Acids.*, 30(3), 279–289.

Hartman, J.W., *et al.* (2007). 'Consumption of fat-free fluid milk after resistance exercise promotes greater lean mass accretion than does consumption of soy or carbohydrate in young, novice, male weightlifters.', *Am. J. Clin. Nutr.*, 86(2), 373–381.

Haub, M.D., *et al.* (1998). 'Acute L-glutamine ingestion does not improve maximal effort exercise.', *J. Sports Med. Phys. Fitness.*, 38(3), 240–244.

Hill, A.M., *et al.* (2007). 'Combining fish-oil supplements with regular aerobic exercise improves body composition and cardiovascular disease risk factors.', *Am. J. Clin. Nutr.*, 85(5), 1267–1274.

Hitchins, S., *et al.* (1999). 'Glycerol hyperhydration improves cycle time trial performance in hot humid conditions.', *Eur. J. Appl. Physiol. Occup. Physiol.*, 80(5), 494–501.

Hobson, R.M., *et al.* (2012). 'Effects of β-alanine supplementation on exercise performance: a meta-analysis.', *Amino Acids.*, 43(1), 25–37.

Hoffman, J.R., *et al.* (2008). 'Short-duration beta-alanine supplementation increases training volume and reduces subjective feelings of fatigue in college football players.', *Nutr. Res.*, 28, 31–35.

Hoon, M.W., et al, (2013) 'The effect of nitrate supplementation on exercise performance in healthy individuals: a systematic review and meta-analysis.' *Int. J. Sports Nutr. Exerc. Metab.*, 23(5): pp. 522–32. (Epub: 2013, Apr. 9).

Hoon M.W., *et al.* (2014). 'Nitrate supplementation and high-intensity performance in competitive cyclists.', *Applied Physiology, Nutrition, and Metabolism*, 0, 0, 10.1139/apnm-2013-0574.

Hord, N.G, Tang, Y., Bryan, N.S. (2009). ' Food sources of nitrates and nitrites: the physiologic context for potential health benefits.', *Am. J. Clin. Nutr.*, 90(1), 1–10.

Howe, S.T., *et al.* (2013). 'The effect of beta-alanine supplementation on isokinetic force and cycling performance in highly trained cyclists.' *Int. J. Sport Nutr. Exerc. Metab.*, 23(6), 562–70.

International Olympic Committee (IOC). (2011). 'Consensus Statement on Sports Nutrition 2010', 4, 29 Suppl 1:S3–4.

International Olympic Committee (IOC). (2011). 'Consensus Statement on Sports Nutrition 2010', Journal of Sports Science, 4 (29) Suppl, 1:S3–4.

Jackman, S.R., *et al.* (2010). 'Branched-chain amino acid ingestion can ameliorate soreness from eccentric exercise.', *Med. Sci. Sports Exerc.* 42(5),962–70.

Jawad, M., *et al.* (2012). 'Safety and Efficacy Profile of Echinacea purpurea to Prevent Common Cold Episodes: A Randomized, Double-Blind, Placebo-Controlled Trial.', *Evidence-Based Complementary and Alternative Medicine.*, vol 2012, Article ID 841315.

Joyce, S., *et al*, (2012) 'Acute and chronic loading of sodium bicarbonate in highly trained swimmers.' *Eur. J. Appl. Physiol.*, 112(2):461-9. doi: 10.1007/s00421-011-1995-z. (Epub: 2011, May 17)

Judkins, C. (2008). 'Investigation into supplementation contamination levels in the UK market', HFL Sport Science. www.informed-sport.com.

Karsch-Völk, M., *et al.* (2014). 'Echinacea for preventing and treating the common cold.' *Cochrane Database Syst Rev.* Feb 20.

Kennerly, K., *et al.* (2011). 'Influence of banana versus sports beverage ingestion on 75 km cycling performance and exercise-induced inflammation', *Med. Sci. Sports Exerc.*, 43(5), 340–341.

King, D.S., *et al.* (1999). 'Effects of oral androstenedione on serum testosterone and adaptations to resistance training in young men', *J. Am. Med. Assoc.*, 281(21), 2020–2028.

Koopman, R., *et al.* (2005). 'Combined ingestion of protein and free leucine with carbohydrate increases postexercise muscle protein synthesis in vivo in male subjects.', *Am. J. Physiol. Endocrinol. Metab.*, 288(4), 645–653.

Kreider, R.B. (2003). 'Effects of creatine supplementation on performance and training adaptations.', *Mol. Cell Biochem.*, 244(1-2), 89–94.

Kreider, R.B., *et al.* (2000). 'Effects of calcium-HMB supplementation during training on markers of catabolism, body composition, strength and sprint performance', *J. Exerc. Physiol.*, 3(4), 48–59.

Lane, S., *et al.* (2013). 'Single and combined effects of beetroot juice and caffeine supplementation on cycling time trial performance', *Appl. Physiol. Nutr. Metab.*, 10.1139/apnm-2013-0336.

Lansley, K.E., *et al.* (2011a). 'Dietary nitrate supplementation reduces the O2 cost of walking and running: a placebo-controlled study', *J. Appl. Physiol.*, 110, 591–600.

Lansley, K.E., *et al.* (2011b). 'Acute dietary nitrate supplementation improves cycling time trial performance', *Med. Sci. Sports Exerc.*, 43, 1125–1131.

Lara, B., *et al.* (2014). 'Caffeine-containing energy drink improves physical performance in female soccer players.', *Amino Acids*, 46(5), 1385–1392.

Larson-Meyer, D.E. and Willis, K.S. (2010). 'Vitamin D and athletes', *Curr Sports Med. Rep.,* 9(4), 220–226.

Lenn, J., *et al.* (2002). 'The effects of fish oil and isoflavones on delayed onset muscle soreness.', *Med. Sci. Sports Exerc.* 34(10), 1605–1613.

Liu, T.H., *et al.* (2009). 'No effect of short-term arginine supplementation on nitric oxide production, metabolism and performance in intermittent exercise in athletes.', *J. Nutr. Biochem.*, 20(6), 462–468.

Lovell, G. (2008). 'Vitamin D status of females in an elite gymnastic programme.', *Clin. J. Sports Med.*, 18, 159–161.

Lugares, R., *et al.* (2013). 'Does long-term creatine supplementation impair kidney function in resistance trained individuals consuming a high protein diet?', *J. Int. Soc. Sports Nutr.* 10, 26.

Lukaski, H.C. (2004). 'Vitamin and mineral status: effects on physical performance.', *Nutrition*, 20, 632–644.

Lun, V., *et al.* (2012). 'Dietary supplementation practices in Canadian high-performance athletes.', *Int. J. Sport Nutr. Exerc. Metab.*, 22(1), 31–37.

MacIntosh, B.R., and Wright, B.M. (1995). 'Caffeine ingestion and performance of a 1,500-metre swim.', *Can. J. Appl. Physiol.*, 20(2), 168–177.

Mackinnon, L.T., and Hooper, S.L. (1996). 'Plasma glutamine and upper respiratory tract infection during intensified training in swimmers.', *Med. Sci. Sports Exerc.*, 28(3), 285–290.

MacLean, D.A., Graham, T.E., and Saltin, B. (1994). 'Branch-chain amino acids augment ammonia metabolism while attenuating protein breakdown during exercise', *Am. J. Physiol.*, 267, 1010–1022.

Maki, K.C., *et al.* (2009). 'Green tea catechin consumption enhances exercise-induced abdominal fat loss in overweight and obese adults.', *J. Nutr.*, 139(2), 264–270.

Mason, W.L., McConell, G., Hargreaves, M. (1993) 'Carbohydrate ingestion during exercise: liquid vs. solid feedings.' *Med. Sci. Sports Exerc.*, 25(8):966–9.

Maughan, R.J., Greenhaff, P.L., and Hespel, P. (2011). 'Dietary supplements for athletes: emerging trends and recurring themes', *J. Sports Sci.*, 29(1), 57–66.

Meier, C., *et al.* (2004). 'Supplementation with oral vitamin D and calcium during winter prevents seasonal bone loss: a randomised controlled open-label prospective trial.', *J. Bone Mineral Res.*, 19, 1221–1230.

MHRA (2012) http://www.mhra.gov.uk/home/groups/comms-po/documents/news/con174847.pdf

Middleton, N., Jelen, P., and Bell, G. (2004). 'Whole blood and mononuclear cell glutathione response to dietary whey protein supplementation in sedentary and trained male human subjects.', *Int. J. Food Sci. Nutr.*, 55(2), 131–141.

Moore, D.R., *et al.* (2009). 'Ingested protein dose response of muscle and albumin protein synthesis after resistance exercise in young men,', *Am. J. Clin. Nutr.*, 89, 161–168.

Murphy, M., *et al.* (2012). 'Whole Beetroot Consumption Acutely Improves Running Performance', *J. Acad. Nutr. Diet*, 112, 548–552.

Nair, K.S., *et al.* (2006). 'DHEA in Elderly Women and DHEA or Testosterone in Elderly Men.', *N. Engl. J. Med.*, 355, 1647–1659.

Neychev, V.K., and Mitev, V.I. (2005). 'The aphrodisiac herb Tribulus terrestris does not influence the androgen production in young men.', *J. Ethnopharmacol.* 101(1–3), 319–2.

Nielsen, F.H., and Lukaski, H.C. (2006). 'Update on the relationship between magnesium and exercise.', *Magnes. Res.*, 19(3), 180–189.

Nieman, D.C., *et al.* (2004). 'Vitamin E and immunity after the Kona Triathlon World Championship.', *Med. Sci. Sports Exerc.*, 36(8), 1328–1335.

Nieman, D.C., *et al* (2012) 'Bananas as an energy source during exercise: a metabolomics approach.' *PLoSONE*, 7(5) e37479.

Nikolaidis, M.G., *et al.* (2012). 'Does vitamin C and E supplementation impair the favorable adaptations of regular exercise?', *Oxid. Med. Cell Longev.* 2012; 2012:707941. doi: 10.1155/2012/707941 (Epub: 2012 Aug 13).

Noakes, T. (2012) 'Waterlogged: The serious problem of overhydration in endurance sports.' *Human Kinetics*.

Noreen, E.E., *et al.* (2010). 'Effects of supplemental fish oil on resting metabolic rate, body composition, and salivary cortisol in healthy adults.', *J. Int. Soc. Sports Nutr.*, 7, 31.

Nosaka, K., Sacco, P., and Mawatari, K. (2006). 'Effects of amino acid supplementation on muscle soreness and damage', *Int. J. Sports Nutr. Exerc. Metab.*, 16, 620–635.

Ostojic, S.M., *et al.* (2007). 'Glucosamine administration in athletes: effects on recovery of acute knee injury.', *Res. Sports Med.* 15(2), 113–124.

Paddon-Jones, D., *et al.* (2001). 'Short term HMB supplementation does not reduce symptoms of eccentric muscle damage', *Int. J. Sport Nutr.*, 11, 442–450.

Parasrampuria, J., Schwartz, K., and Petesch, R. (1998). 'Quality Control of Dehydroepiandrosterone Dietary Supplement Products.', *JAMA.*, 280(18), 1565.

Pasiakos, S.M., McClung, H.L., and McClung, J.P. (2011). 'Leucine-enriched essential amino acid supplementation during moderate steady state exercise enhances postexercise muscle protein synthesis.', *Am. J. Clin. Nutr.*, 94(3), 809–818.

Pasiakos, S.M., and McClung, J.P. (2011). 'Supplemental dietary leucine and the skeletal muscle anabolic response to essential amino acids.', *Nutr. Rev.*, 69(9), 550–557.

Pasricha, S.R., *et al.* (2014). 'Iron Supplementation Benefits Physical Performance in Women of Reproductive Age: A Systematic Review and Meta-Analysis.', *J. Nutr.* 2014 jn.113.189589; first published online April 9, 2014.

Patterson, S.D., and Gray, S.C. (2007). 'Carbohydrate-gel supplementation and endurance performance during intermittent high-intensity shuttle running', *Int. J. Sports Nutr. Exerc. Metab.*, 17, 445–455.

Paulsen, G., *et al.* (2013). 'Vitamin C and E supplementation hampers cellular adaptation to endurance training in humans: a double-blind randomized controlled trial.', *J. Physiol.* 2013.267419.

Peternelj, T.T., and Coombes, J.S. (2011). 'Antioxidant supplementation during exercise training: beneficial or detrimental?', *Sports Med.*, 1;41(12), 1043–1069.

Peters, E.M., *et al.* (1993). 'Vitamin C supplementation reduces the incidence of post-race symptoms of upper-respiratory-tract infection in ultra-marathon runners', *Am. J. Clin. Nutr.*, 57, 170–174.

Peters, E.M., *et al.* (2001). 'Vitamin C supplementation attenuates the increases in circulating cortisol, adrenaline and anti-inflammatory polypeptides following ultra-marathon running', *Int. J. Sports Med.*, 22(7), 537–543.

Pfeiffer, B., *et al.* (2010). 'CHO oxidation from a CHO gel compared with a drink during exercise.', *Med. Sci. Sports Exerc.*, 42(11), 2038–2045.

Phillips, G.C. (2007). 'Glutamine: the nonessential amino acid for performance enhancement.', *Curr Sports Med. Rep.*, 6(4), 265–268.

Phillips, M.D., *et al.* (2013). 'Pre-exercise energy drink consumption does not improve endurance cycling performance, but increases lactate, monocyte and IL-6 response.', *J. Strength Cond. Res.* Oct 29. (Epub ahead of print).

Phillips, S.M., *et al.* (2007). 'A critical examination of dietary protein requirements, benefits and excesses in athletes', *Int. J. Sports Nutr. Exerc. Metab.,* 17, 58–78.

Phillips, S.M. and Van Loon, L. J. (2011), 'Dietary protein for athletes: from requirements to optimum adaptation' *J. Sports Sci.*, vol. 29, Suppl 1:S29–38.

Phillips, T., *et al.* (2003). 'A dietary supplement attenuates IL-6 and CRP after eccentric exercise in untrained males.', *Med. Sci. Sports Exerc.* 35(12), 2032–2037.

Pollock, N., *et al.* (2012). 'Low 25(OH) vitamin D concentrations in international UK track and field athletes.', *S. Afr. J. Sports Med.,* 24(2), 55–59.

Poolsup, N., *et al.* (2005). 'Glucosamine long-term treatment and the progression of knee osteoarthritis: systematic review of randomized controlled trials.', *Ann. Pharmacother.,* 39(6), 1080–1087.

Powers, M.E. (2002). 'The safety and efficacy of anabolic steroid precursors: What is the scientific evidence?', *J. Athletic Training,* 37(3), 300–305.

Powers, S., Nelson, W.B., and Larson-Meyer, E. (2011). 'Antioxidant and vitamin D supplements for athletes: sense or nonsense?', *J. Sports Sci.,* 29 (1), 47–55.

Quesnele, J.J., *et al.* (2004). 'The effects of Beta-alanine supplementation on performance: a systematic review of the literature.', *Int. J. Sport Nutr. Exerc. Metab.,* 24(1), 14–27.

Rawson, E.S., and Volek, J.S. (2003). 'Effects of creatine supplementation and resistance training on muscle strength and weightlifting performance.', *J. Strength Cond. Res.,* 17, 822–831.

Res, P.T., *et al.* (2012). 'Protein ingestion before sleep improves post-exercise overnight recovery,', *Med. Sci. Sports Exerc.,* 44(8), 1560–1569.

Rizos, E.C., *et al.* (2012). 'Association Between Omega-3 Fatty Acid

Supplementation and Risk of Major Cardiovascular Disease Events: A Systematic Review and Meta-analysis.', *JAMA.*, 308(10), 1024–1033.

American Dietetic Association; Dietitians of Canada; American College of Sports Medicine; Rodriguez, N.R., *et al.* (2009). 'American College of Sports Medicine position stand: Nutrition and athletic performance.', *Med. Sci. Sports Exerc.*, 41(3), 709–731.

Rogerson, S., *et al.* (2007). 'The effect of five weeks of Tribulus terrestris supplementation on muscle strength and body composition during preseason training in elite rugby league players.', *J. Strength Cond. Res.*, 21(2), 348–353.

Rokitzki, L., *et al.* (1994). 'A-tocopherol supplementation in racing cyclists during extreme endurance training', *Int. J. Sports Nutr.*, 4, 235–264.

Rowlands, D.S., and Thomson, J.S. (2009). 'Effects of beta-hydroxy-beta-methylbutyrate supplementation during resistance training on strength, body composition, and muscle damage in trained and untrained young men: a meta-analysis.', *J. Strength Cond. Res.*, 23(3), 836–846.

Rowlands, D.S., *et al.* (2012). 'Composite versus single transportable carbohydrate solution enhances race and laboratory cycling performance.', *Appl. Physiol. Nutr. Metab.*, 37, 425–436.

Rowlands, D.S., *et al.* (2008). 'Effect of graded fructose co-ingestion with maltodextrin on exogenous 14C-fructose and 13C-glucose oxidation efficiency and high-intensity cycling performance.', *J. Appl. Physiol.*, 104, 1709–1719.

Russell, C., Hall, D., and Brown, P. (2013). *European Supplement Contamination Survey*, www.informed-sport.com.

Rutherford, J.A., Spriet, L.L., and Stellingwerff, T. (2010). 'The effect of acute taurine ingestion on endurance performance and metabolism in well-trained cyclists.', *Int. J. Sport Nutr. Exerc. Metab.*, 20(4), 322–329.

Sale, C., Saunders B., and Harris, R.C. (2010). 'Effect of beta-alanine supplementation on muscle carnosine concentrations and exercise performance.', *Amino Acids* 39, 321–333.

Santos, V.C., *et al.* (2013). 'Effects of DHA-rich fish oil supplementation on lymphocyte function before and after a marathon race.', *Int. J. Sport Nutr. Exerc. Metab.*, 23(2), 161–169.

Shimomura, Y., *et al.* (2010). 'Branched-chain amino acid supplementation before squat exercise and delayed-onset muscle soreness.', *Int. J. Sport Nutr. Exerc. Metab.*, 20(3), 236-244.

Shing, C.M., *et al.* (2007). 'Effects of bovine colostrum supplementation on immune variables in highly trained cyclists.', *J. Appl. Physiol.*, 102, 1113–1122.

Shing, C.M., Hunter, D.C., and Stevenson, L.M. (2009). 'Bovine colostrum supplementation and exercise performance: potential mechanisms.', *Sports Med.* 39(12), 1033–1054.

Shirreffs, S.M., Watson, P., and Maughan, R.J. (2007). 'Milk as an effective post-exercise rehydration drink.', *British Journal of Nutrition,* 1-8.

Shirreffs, S.M., and Sawka, M.N. (2011). 'Fluid and electrolyte needs for training, competition, and recovery.', *J. Sports. Sci.,* 29(1), 39–46.

Silva, A.M., *et al.* (2013). 'Total body water and its compartments are not affected by ingesting a moderate dose of caffeine in healthy young adult males.', *Appl. Physiol. Nutr. Metab.,* 38, 626-632.

Skaug, A., Sveen, O., and Raastad, T. (2014). 'An antioxidant and multivitamin supplement reduced improvements in VO_2max', *J. Sports. Med. Physical Fitness*, 54(1), 63-69.

Slater, G., *et al.* (2001). 'Beta-hydroxy-beta-methylbutyrate (HMB) supplementation does not affect changes in strength or body composition during resistance training in trained men', *Int. J. Sport Nutr.*, 11, 383–396.

Smith, J.W., *et al.* (2013). 'Curvilinear dose-response relationship of carbohydrate (0-120 g·h(-1)) and performance.', *Med. Sci. Sports Exerc.*, 45(2),336–341.

Smith, W.A., *et al.* (2008). 'Effect of glycine propionyl-L-carnitine on aerobic and anaerobic exercise performance.', *Int. J. Sport Nutr. Exerc. Metab.,* 18(1), 19-36.

Stegen, S., *et al*. (2014). 'The Beta-Alanine Dose for Maintaining Moderately Elevated Muscle Carnosine Levels.', *Med. Sci. Sports Exerc*. 1. (Epub ahead of print).

Tang, J.E., *et al*. (2009). 'Ingestion of whey hydrolysate, casein, or soy protein isolate: effects on mixed muscle protein synthesis at rest and following resistance exercise in young men.', *J. Appl. Physiol*., 107(3), 987–992.

Temesi, J., *et al*. (2011). 'Carbohydrate ingestion during endurance exercise improves performance in adults.', *J. Nutr.*, 41(5), 890–987.

Theodorou, A.A., *et al*. (2011). 'No effect of antioxidant supplementation on muscle performance and blood redox status adaptations to eccentric training.' *Am. J. Clin. Nutr.*, 93(6), 1373–1383.

Tipton, K.D., *et al*. (2004). 'Ingestion of casein and whey proteins result in muscle anabolism after resistance exercise.', *Med. Sci. Sports Exerc.*, 36(12), 2073–2081.

Too, B., *et al*. (2012). 'Natural versus commercial carbohydrate supplementation and endurance running performance.', *J. Int. Soc. Sports Nutr.*, 9, 27.

Transparency Market Research. (2014). 'Sports Nutrition Market – Global Industry Analysis, Size, Share, Growth, Trends and Forecast, 2013–2019', www.transparencymarketresearch.com/sports-nutrition-market.html.

Trappe, S.W., *et al*. (1994). 'The effects of L-carnitine supplementation on performance during interval swimming.', *Int. J. Sports Med.*, 15(4), 181–185.

Triplett, D., *et al*. (2010). 'An isocaloric glucose fructose beverage's effect on simulated 100-km cycling performance compared with a glucose-only beverage.', *Int. J. Sport Nutr. Exerc. Metab.*, 20, 122-131.

Troesch, B., *et al*. (2012). 'Dietary surveys indicate vitamin intakes below recommendations are common in representative Western countries.', *Brit. J. Nutr.*, 108:4, 692–698.

Vandenbogaerde, T. J., and Hopkins, W.G. (2011). 'Effects of Acute Carbohydrate Supplementation on Endurance Performance: A Meta-Analysis', *Sports Medicine*, 41(9), 773–792.

Van Rosendal, S.P., *et al.* (2009). 'Physiological and performance effects of glycerol hyperhydration and rehydration.', *Nutr. Rev.*, 67(12), 690–705.

Van Rosendal, S.P., *et al.* (2010). 'Guidelines for glycerol use in hyperhydration and rehydration associated with exercise.', *Sports Med.*, 40(2), 113–129.

Van Thienen, R., *et al.* (2009). 'Beta-alanine improves sprint performance in endurance cycling.', *Med. Sci. Sports Exerc.*, 41, 898–903.

Venables, M.C., *et al.* (2008). 'Green tea extract ingestion, fat oxidation, and glucose tolerance in healthy humans.' *Am. J. Clin. Nutr.*, 87(3), 778–784.

Villacis, D., *et al.* (2014). 'Prevalence of Abnormal Vitamin D Levels Among Division I NCAA Athletes.', *Sports Health: A Multidisciplinary Approach.*

Villani, R.G., *et al.* (2000). 'L-Carnitine supplementation combined with aerobic training does not promote weight loss in moderately obese women.', *Int. J. Sport Nutr. Exerc. Metab.*, 10(2), 199–207.

WADA (2014) 'The 2014 Prohibited List.' www.wada-ama.org/en/Science-Medicine/Prohibited-List/

Wallace, M.B., *et al.* (1999). 'Effects of dehydroepiandrosterone vs androstenedione supplementation in men.', *Med. Sci. Sports Exerc.* 31(12), 1788–1792.

Wallis, G.A., *et al.* (2005). 'Oxidation of combined ingestion of maltodextrins and fructose during exercise.', *Med. Sci. Sports Exerc.*, 37, 426–432.

Walser, B., Giordano, R.M., and Stebbins, C.L. (2006). 'Supplementation with omega-3 polyunsaturated fatty acids augments brachial artery dilation and blood flow during forearm contraction.', *Eur. J. Appl. Physiol.*, 97(3), 347–354.

Wandel, S., *et al.* (2010). 'Effects of glucosamine, chondroitin, or placebo in patients with osteoarthritis of hip or knee: network meta-analysis', *BMJ*, 341, 4675.

Weisgarber, K.D., Candow, D.G., and Vogt, E.S.M. (2012). 'Whey Protein Before and During Resistance Exercise Has No Effect on

Muscle Mass and Strength in Untrained Young Adults.', *Int. J. Sport Nutr. Exerc. Metab.*

West, N.P., *et al.* (2011). 'Supplementation with Lactobacillus fermentum VRI (PCC) reduces lower respiratory illness in athletes and moderate exercise-induced immune perturbations.', *Nutrition Journal.*, 10, 30.

Wiens, K., *et al.* (2014). 'Dietary Supplement Usage, Motivation, and Education in Young, Canadian Athletes.' *Int. J. Sport Nutr. Exerc. Metab.* (Epub ahead of print).

Wilborn, C.D., *et al.* (2004). 'Effects of Zinc Magnesium Aspartate (ZMA) Supplementation on Training Adaptations and Markers of Anabolism and Catabolism.', *J. Int. Soc. Sports Nutr.*, 1(2), 12–20.

Wilkinson, S.B., *et al.* (2007). 'Consumption of fluid skim milk promotes greater protein accretion after resistance exercise than does consumption of an isonitrogenous and isoenergetic soy-protein beverage,', *Am. J. Clin. Nutr.*, 85(4), 1031–1040.

Willoughby, D.S., *et al.* (2007). 'Effects of resistance training and protein plus amino acid supplementation on muscle anabolism, mass, and strength.' *Amino Acids.*, 32(4), 467–477.

Willoughby, D.S., *et al.* (2011). 'Effects of 7 days of arginine-alpha-ketoglutarate supplementation on blood flow, plasma L-arginine, nitric oxide metabolites, and asymmetric dimethyl arginine after resistance exercise.', *Int. J. Sport Nutr. Exerc. Metab.*, 21(4), 291–299.

Wilson, J.M., *et al.* (2013). 'International Society of Sports Nutrition Position Stand: beta-hydroxy-beta-methylbutyrate (HMB)', *J. Int. Soc. Sports Nutr.*, 10(1), 6.

Wylie, L.J., *et al* (2013) 'Beetroot juice and exercise: pharmacodynamic and dose-response relationships.' *J. Appl. Physiol.* May 2 [Epub ahead of print]

Yaspelkis, B.B., *et al.* (1993) 'Carbohydrate supplementation spares muscle glycogen during variable-intensity exercise.' J. Appl. Physiol. Oct; 75(4):1477–85.

Yfanti, C., *et al.* (2010). 'Antioxidant supplementation does not alter endurance training adaptation.', *Med. Sci. Sports Exerc.*, 42(7), 1388–1395.

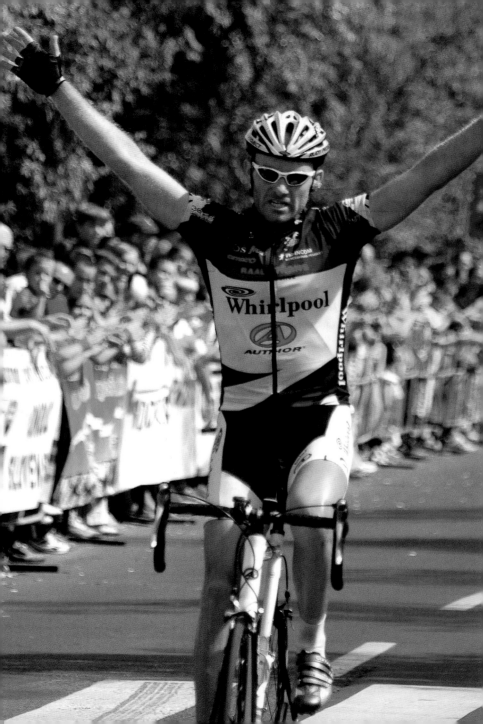

RESOURCES

SPORT AND EXERCISE NUTRITION WEBSITES

www.associationfornutrition.org (provides a register of UK nutritionists specialising in sport)

www.scandpg.org/sports-nutrition (Sports Dietetics-USA, a subgroup of the Academy of Nutrition and Dietetics)

www.sportsdietitians.org.uk (Sports Dietitians UK, a sub-group of the British Dietetic Association)

www.acsm.org (The American College of Sports Medicine)

www.ausport.gov.au/ais/nutrition (The Sports Nutrition group of the Australian Institute of Sport)

www.sportsrd.org (The Collegiate and Professional Sports Dietitians Association)

www.ncaa.org (The National Collegiate Athletic Association)

www.nsca.com (The National Strength and Conditioning Association)

www.sportsdietitians.com.au (Sports Dietitians Australia)

www.teamusa.org (United States Olympic Committee)

INFORMATION ON BANNED DRUGS: EDUCATION, RULES, AND TESTING

www.wada-ama.org (World Anti-Doping Agency, WADA)

www.ukad.org.uk (UK Anti-Doping, UKAD)

www.usantidoping.org (US Anti-Doping Agency, USADA)

www.informed-sport.com (Informed Sport, a quality assurance programme for sports supplements) www.ncaa.org/health-and-safety/policy/2013-14-ncaa-banned-drugs (The NCAA Banned Drug List)

http://www.nsfsport.com (The NSF Certified for Sport® Program)

www.supplementsafetynow.com (Supplement Safety Now, a public protection initiative founded by the US Anti-Doping Agency)

www.drugfreesport.com (The US National Center for Drug Free Sport)

www.consumerlab.com (ConsumerLab, an independent testing organisation for nutritional products)

www.usp.org (US Pharmacopeia Dietary Supplement Verification Program)

TO FIND A SPORT AND EXERCISE NUTRITIONIST

http://www.associationfornutrition.org/ (the UK Voluntary Register of Nutritionists)

www.senr.org.uk (the voluntary competency based register for Sport and Exercise Nutritionists)

www.scandpg.org/search-rd (a register for dietitians specialising in sport nutrition in the US)

INDEX